Textbook of Microbiology

for Diploma in General Nursing and Midwifery Students

Textbook of Microbiology
for Diploma in General Nursing and Midwifery Students

Second Edition

Surinder Kumar
MD DNB MNAMS
Director Professor (Ex)
Department of Microbiology
Maulana Azad Medical College
New Delhi, India

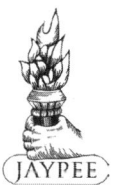

JAYPEE BROTHERS MEDICAL PUBLISHERS
The Health Sciences Publisher
New Delhi | London

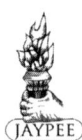

Jaypee Brothers Medical Publishers (P) Ltd

Headquarters

Jaypee Brothers Medical Publishers (P) Ltd
EMCA House, 23/23-B
Ansari Road, Daryaganj
New Delhi 110 002, India
Landline: +91-11-23272143, +91-11-23272703
+91-11-23282021, +91-11-23245672
Email: jaypee@jaypeebrothers.com

Corporate Office

Jaypee Brothers Medical Publishers (P) Ltd
4838/24, Ansari Road, Daryaganj
New Delhi 110 002, India
Phone: +91-11-43574357
Fax: +91-11-43574314
Email: jaypee@jaypeebrothers.com

Overseas Office

J.P. Medical Ltd
83 Victoria Street, London
SW1H 0HW (UK)
Phone: +44 20 3170 8910
Fax: +44 (0)20 3008 6180
Email: info@jpmedpub.com

Website: www.jaypeebrothers.com
Website: www.jaypeedigital.com

© 2023, Jaypee Brothers Medical Publishers

The views and opinions expressed in this book are solely those of the original contributor(s)/author(s) and do not necessarily represent those of editor(s) and publisher of the book.

All rights reserved. No part of this publication may be reproduced, stored or transmitted in any form or by any means, electronic, mechanical, photocopying, recording or otherwise, without the prior permission in writing of the publishers.

All brand names and product names used in this book are trade names, service marks, trademarks or registered trademarks of their respective owners. The publisher is not associated with any product or vendor mentioned in this book.

Medical knowledge and practice change constantly. This book is designed to provide accurate, authoritative information about the subject matter in question. However, readers are advised to check the most current information available on procedures included and check information from the manufacturer of each product to be administered, to verify the recommended dose, formula, method and duration of administration, adverse effects and contraindications. It is the responsibility of the practitioner to take all appropriate safety precautions. Neither the publisher nor the author(s)/editor(s) assume any liability for any injury and/or damage to persons or property arising from or related to use of material in this book.

This book is sold on the understanding that the publisher is not engaged in providing professional medical services. If such advice or services are required, the services of a competent medical professional should be sought.

Every effort has been made where necessary to contact holders of copyright to obtain permission to reproduce copyright material. If any have been inadvertently overlooked, the publisher will be pleased to make the necessary arrangements at the first opportunity.

Inquiries for bulk sales may be solicited at: jaypee@jaypeebrothers.com

Textbook of Microbiology for Diploma in General Nursing and Midwifery Students

First Edition: 2016

Second Edition: **2023**

ISBN: 978-93-5465-913-3

Printed at: Sterling Graphics Pvt. Ltd. India.

Dedicated to

My Father
Late Shri Lachhman Das

My Mother
Late Smt Bal Kaur

My Wife
Dr (Prof) Savita Kumari

and

My Sons
Dr Sourabh Kumar and Sanchit Kumar
Whose love and energy make everything I do possible.

Preface to the Second Edition

Students have been using *Textbook of Microbiology for Diploma in General Nursing and Midwifery Students* as readable and complete enough to meet their needs with complete coverage of subject since the publication of the first edition. There are many ways to approach learning microbiology, but ultimately the more you interact with the material using multiple senses, the better you will build memory and learn. I used my experience as an author and teacher to choose the most important information and explanations for inclusion in this textbook. This book remains true to the goals of the first edition to provide a brief, accurate and up-to-date presentation with limited time and the latest syllabus. These aims are achieved by using several different formats, which should make the book useful to students with varying study objectives and learning styles. This book is divided into six sections (Introduction, Microorganisms, Infection and its Transmission, Immunology, The Control and Destruction of Microorganisms, and Introduction to Laboratory Techniques) and twenty chapters based on syllabus of microbiology for Diploma in General Nursing and Midwifery. Each chapter has been carefully updated and in each of these chapters, I have attempted to present the material that will help the student gain an interest and a clear understanding of the subject. I hope second edition of book meets the criteria that presents the most important information and explanations in a readable, interesting, and varied format. I shall be thankful for any comment or suggestions from students, teachers and all the readers of this book for further improvement.

Surinder Kumar

Preface to the First Edition

Microbiology is an inherently valuable and useful discipline that offers an intimate view of an invisible world and can be a bewildering field to the novice. Traditional books are too long and detailed to be read by the student who is trying to keep up with several classes simultaneously of other subjects. *Textbook of Microbiology for Diploma in General Nursing and Midwifery Students* has been written after 28 years of teaching medical, dental and nursing students, and after searching for a book that was both readable and complete enough to meet the needs of the students of diploma in general nursing and midwifery. The book contains all of the information that are pertinent to students who are studying microbiology keeping in mind their examination. The orientation of the book continues to be a presentation that is understandable to students of diverse backgrounds.

The book is divided into 6 sections, based on the major disciplines included within syllabus in microbiology for diploma in general nursing and midwifery such as introduction, microorganisms, infection and its transmission, immunity, control and destruction of microorganisms and introduction to laboratory techniques. The chapters themselves are comprehensive yet free of unnecessary detail and provide the reader with a framework for understanding. I hope that the book will be received with enthusiasm and will fulfill the needs of diploma in general nursing and midwifery students. I shall be thankful for any comment or suggestions from students, teachers and all the readers of the book for further improvement.

Surinder Kumar

Acknowledgments

I am grateful to all teachers, students, instructors, and many other individuals, who have all made invaluable suggestions and comments on ways to improve this second edition of *Textbook of Microbiology For Diploma in General Nursing and Midwifery Students*. I am thankful to the whole team of M/s Jaypee Brothers Medical Publishers (P) Ltd, New Delhi, India, who helped and guided me, Shri Jitendar P Vij (Group Chairman), Mr Ankit Vij (Managing Director), Mr MS Mani (Group President), Dr Madhu Choudhary (Director-Educational Publishing), Ms Pooja Bhandari (Production Head), Ms Sunita Katla (Executive Assistant to Group Chairman and Publishing Manager), Ms Samina Khan (Executive Assistant to Director-Educational Publishing), Mr Rajesh Sharma (Production Coordinator), Ms Seema Dogra (Cover Visualizer), Ms Geeta Barik (Proofreader), Mr Kulwant Singh (Typesetter), Mr Nitin Bhardwaj (Graphic Designer) and their team members, for all their support to work in this project and make it a success.

I am especially grateful to my wife Dr Savita Kumari, my sons Dr Sourabh Kumar and Dr Sanchit Kumar for their support, invaluable help and understanding in making this book a reality.

Contents

Section 1: Introduction

Chapter 1: Historical Development of Microbiology   3
- Introduction and Scope *3*
- Infection and Contagion *3*
- Discovery of Microorganisms *4*
- The Conflict Over Spontaneous Generation *4*
- Role of Microorganisms in Disease *5*
- Scientific Development of Microbiology *5*
- Discovery of Viruses *9*
- Serotherapy and Chemotherapy *9*
- Branches of Microbiology *10*
- Scope of Microbiology in Nursing *10*
- Nobel Prizes Awarded for Research in Microbiology *12*

Section 2: Microorganisms

Chapter 2: Morphology of Bacteria   19
- Naming and Classifying Microorganisms *19*
- Study of Bacteria *21*
- Anatomy of the Bacterial Cell *24*

Chapter 3: Physiology of Bacteria   37
- Principles of Bacterial Growth *37*

Chapter 4: Normal Microbial Flora of the Human Body   43
- Normal Flora of the Skin *43*
- Normal Flora of the Conjunctiva *43*
- Normal Flora of the Nose, Nasopharynx and Accessory Sinuses *44*
- Normal Flora of the Mouth *44*
- Normal Flora of the Upper Respiratory Tract *44*
- Normal Flora of the Gastrointestinal Tract *45*
- Normal Flora of the Genitourinary Tract *45*

Chapter 5: Pathogenesis and Common Diseases   48
- Common Diseases Caused by Different Microorganisms *18*
- Human Diseases Caused by Bacteria *48*
- Human Diseases Caused by Fungi *53*
- Human Diseases Caused by Parasites *55*
- Viruses *56*

Chapter 6: Methods for Study of Microbes — 62
- Methods for Study of Microbes *62*

Chapter 7: Culture Media and Culture Methods — 68
- Classification of Media *68*
- Culture Methods *74*

Section 3: Infection and its Transmission

Chapter 8: Infection and Asepsis — 81
- Factors Predisposing to Microbial Pathogenicity *87*
- Asepsis *90*

Chapter 9: Collection of Specimens — 93
- Specimens *93*
- Universal Precautions *94*
- Collection *94*
- Transport of Specimens *99*
- Health and Safety Precautions *99*

Section 4: Immunology

Chapter 10: Immunity — 103
- Classification *103*
- Mechanisms of Innate Immunity *104*
- Types of Immunity *105*

Chapter 11: Immunoprophylaxis — 111
- Immunizing Agents *111*
- Immunization *114*

Chapter 12: Hypersensitivity Reactions — 121
- Hypersensitivity *121*
- Classification of Hypersensitivity Reactions *121*

Chapter 13: Autoimmunity — 132
- Mechanisms of Autoimmunity *132*
- Classification of Autoimmune Diseases *133*

Chapter 14: Principles and Uses of Serological Tests — 135
- Serologic Diagnosis *135*

Section 5: The Control and Destruction of Microorganisms

Chapter 15: Sterilization and Disinfection — 149
- Methods of Sterilization and Disinfection *149*
- Recommended Concentrations of Disinfectants Commonly Used in the Hospitals *164*
- Cleaning *165*
- Asepsis *166*
- Spaulding's Classification *167*

Chapter 16: Antimicrobial Chemotherapy — 172
- Antibacterial Agents *173*
- Mechanisms of Action of Antibacterial Drugs *174*
- Resistance to Antimicrobial Drugs *177*

Chapter 17: Biomedical Waste Management — 179
- Biomedical Waste Management in India *188*
- Laundry Management Process *190*

Section 6: Introduction to Laboratory Techniques

Chapter 18: Microscopy — 195
- Microscopy: Instruments *195*
- Care of the Microscope *200*

Chapter 19: Staining Methods — 203
- Methods of Staining *207*
- Common Staining Techniques *208*
- Methods for Detection for Direct Microscopic Detection of Fungi in Clinical Specimens *217*

Chapter 20: Identification of Common Microbes under the Microscope — 219
- Examination Methods *219*
- Examination of Prepared Material *223*
- Search for Microorganisms *223*

Index — *225*

GNM Syllabus

MICROBIOLOGY

Course Description

This course is designed to help students gain knowledge and understanding of the characteristics and activities of microorganisms, how they react under different conditions and how they cause different disorders and diseases. Knowledge of these principles will enable student to understand and adopt practices associated with preventive and promotive health care.

General Objectives

Upon completion of the course, the students shall be able to:
- Describe the classifications and characteristics of microorganisms.
- List the common disease producing microorganisms.
- Explain the activities of microorganism in relation to the environment and the human body.
- Enumerate the basic principles of control and destruction of microorganisms.
- Apply the principles of microbiology in nursing practice.

Total hours – 30

Unit. No.	Learning objectives	Content	Hours	Teaching/ learning activities	Assessment methods
I	Describe evolution of microbiology and its relevance in nursing.	Introduction a. History of bacteriology and microbiology b. Scope of microbiology in nursing	3	Lecture-cum-discussions	Objective type Short answers
II	Classify the different types of micro organism. Describe the normal flora and the common diseases caused by pathogens. Explain the methods to study microbes.	**Microorganisms** a. Classification, characteristics, (structure, size, method and rate of reproduction) b. Normal flora of the body c. Pathogenesis and common diseases d. Methods for study of microbes, culture and isolation of microbes	8	Lecture-cum-discussions Explain using slides, films, videos, exhibits, models Staining and fixation of slides.	Short answer Objective type Essay type
III	Describe the sources of infection and growth of microbes. Explain the transmission of infection and the principles in collecting specimens.	**Infection and its transmission** a. Sources and types of infection, nosocomial infection b. Factors affecting growth of microbes c. Cycle of transmission of infection portals of entry, exit, modes of transfer d. Reaction of body to infection, mechanism of resistance e. Collection of specimens	4	Lecture Demonstrations specimens Explain using charts	Short answer Objective type Essay type

GNM Syllabus

Unit. No.	Learning objectives	Content	Hrours	Teaching/ learning activities	Assessment methods
IV	Describe various types of immunity, hypersensitivity autoimmunity and immunizing agents.	**Immunity** a. Types of immunity – innate and acquired. b. Immunization schedule. c. Immunoprophylaxis (vaccines, sera etc.) d. Hypersensitivity and autoimmunity. e. Principles and uses of serological tests	5	Lecture-cum-discussions Demonstration exhibits	Short answer Objective type Essay type

V	Describe the various methods of control and destruction of microbes.	**Control and destruction of microbes**
		a. Principles and methods of microbial control
		  – Sterilization
		  – Disinfection
		  – Chemotherapy and antibiotics
		  – Pasteurization
		b. Medical and surgical asepsis
		c. Bio-safety and waste management
			5	Lecture,
				Demonstration
				Videos Visit to the CSSD
					Short answer
					Objective type
					Essay type

VI.	Demonstrate skill in handling and care of microscopes. Identify common microbes under the microscope	**Practical microbiology** a. Microscope–parts, uses, handling and care of microscope b. Observation of staining procedure, preparation and examination of slides and smears c. Identification of common microbes under the microscope for morphology of different microbes.	5	Lecture, Demonstrations Specimens Slides	

Plate 1

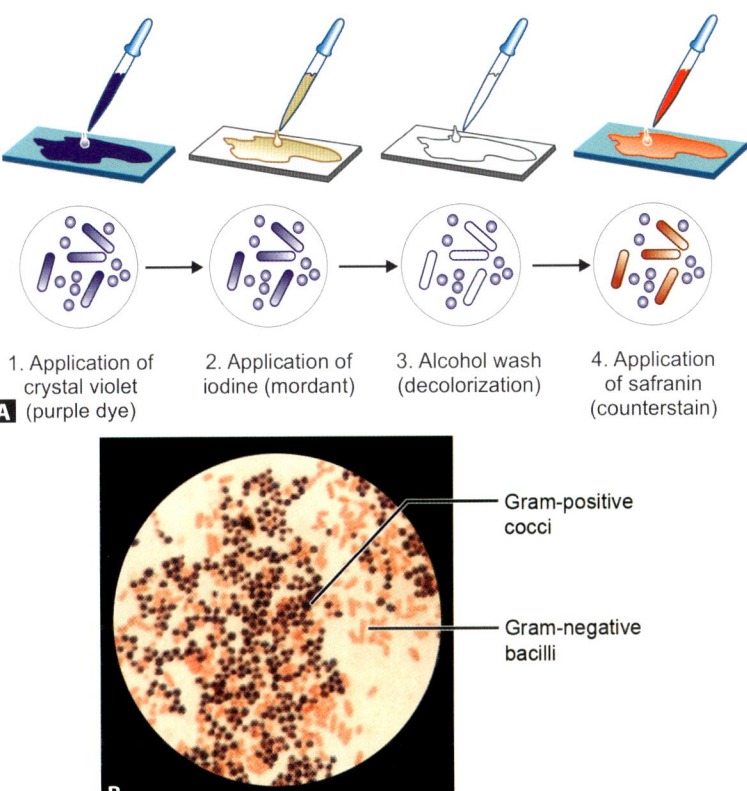

Figs. 19.3A and B: Gram stain: (A) Steps in the Gram stain procedure; (B) Results of a Gram stain. The Gram-positive cells (purple) are *Staphylococcus aureus*; the Gram-negative cells (reddish-pink) are *Escherichia coli*.

Plate 2

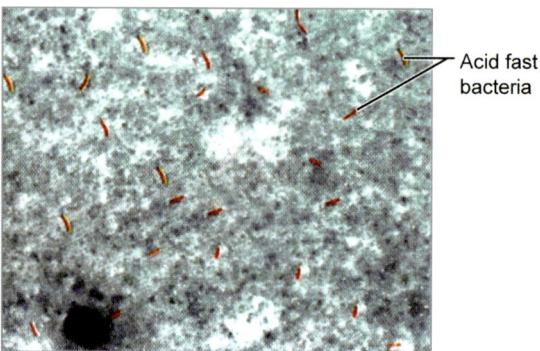

Fig. 19.4: Ziehl-Neelsen stain (100X).

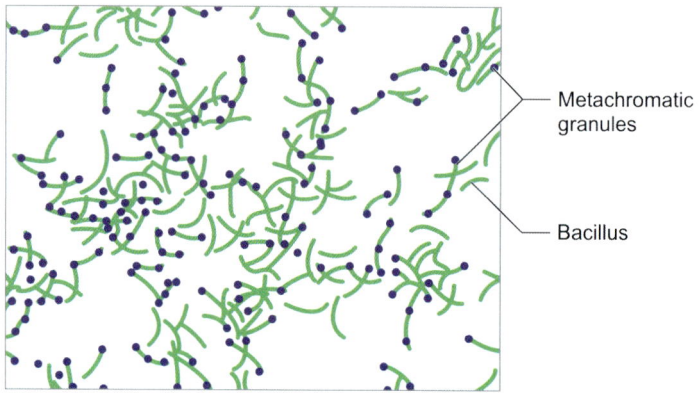

Fig. 19.5: Albert's stain (100X).

SECTION 1

Introduction

Section Outline

- ❖ Historical Development of Microbiology

CHAPTER 1

Historical Development of Microbiology

Learning Objectives

After reading and studying this chapter, you should be able to:
1. Describe the following:
   a. Contributions of Antony van Leeuwenhoek.
   b. Contributions of Louis Pasteur.
   c. Contributions of Robert Koch.
   d. Koch's postulates.
2. Explain concepts and principles of microbiology and their importance in nursing.

■ INTRODUCTION AND SCOPE

Microbiology is the study of living organisms of microscopic size. **Medical microbiology** is the subdivision concerned with the causative agents of infectious disease of man, the response of the host to infection and various methods of diagnosis, treatment, and prevention. The term microbe was first used by Sedillot in 1878, but now is commonly replaced by microorganisms.

■ INFECTION AND CONTAGION

Ancient belief: Among ancient peoples, epidemic and even endemic diseases were believed to be supernatural in origin, sent by the Gods as punishment for the sins of human kind.

Concept of contagion: Long before microbes had been seen, observations on communicable diseases had given rise to the concept of contagion: the spread of disease by contact, direct or indirect.

Invisible living creatures produced disease: Varro in the second century BC later recorded the principle of contagion by invisible creatures. **Roger Bacon**, in the thirteenth century postulated that invisible living creatures produced disease.

■ DISCOVERY OF MICROORGANISMS

First Observation of Microorganisms

As microbes are invisible to the unaided eye, direct observation of microorganisms had to await the development of the microscope.

Antony van Leeuwenhoek (1632–1723)

The credit for having first observed and reported bacteria belongs to Antony van Leeuwenhoek. Antony van Leeuwenhoek, the Dutchman, was a draper and haberdasher in Delft, Holland. He was the amateur microscopist and was the first person to observe microorganisms (1673) using a simple microscope. In 1683, he made accurate descriptions of various types of bacteria and communicated them to the Royal Society of London. Their importance in medicine and in other areas of biology came to be recognized two centuries later.

■ THE CONFLICT OVER SPONTANEOUS GENERATION

Spontaneous Generation (Abiogenesis)

From earliest times, people had believed in **spontaneous generation (abiogenesis)** that living organisms could develop from nonliving matter.

i. **Evidence pro:** Some proposed that microorganisms arose by spontaneous generation though larger organisms did not.

ii. **Evidence con—the spontaneous generation experiment:** **Lazzaro Spallanzani (1729-1799)**, an Italian priest and naturalist opposed this view, who boiled beef broth for an hour, sealed the flasks, and observed no formation of microbes. **Franz Schulze (1815-1873), Theodore Schwann (1810-1882), Georg Friedrich Schroder** and **Theodor von Dusch**—attempted to counter such arguments. **Louis Pasteur (1822-1895)** settled this matter once and for all.

ROLE OF MICROORGANISMS IN DISEASE

A firm basis for the casual nature of infectious disease was established only in the latter half of the nineteenth century. Fungi, being larger than bacteria, were the first agents to be recognized **Agostino Bassi (1773–1856)** demonstrated in 1835 that a silkworm disease called muscardine was due to a fungal infection. **MJ Berkeley (1845)** proved that the great potato blight of Ireland was caused by a fungus. Following his success with the study of fermentation, Pasteur was asked by French government to investigate the **pebrine disease of silkworm** that was disrupting the silk industry. He showed that the disease was due to a protozoan parasite after several years of work.

SCIENTIFIC DEVELOPMENT OF MICROBIOLOGY

The development of microbiology as a scientific discipline from era of Louis Pasteur, perfection on microbiological studies by Robert Koch, the introduction of antiseptic surgery by Lord Lister and contributions of Paul Ehrlich in chemotherapy.

Louis Pasteur (1822–1895)

Louis Pasteur (1822-1895) was born in the village of Dole, France on December 27, 1822 the son of humble parents **(Fig. 1.1)**. He was originally trained as a chemist, but his studies on fermentation led

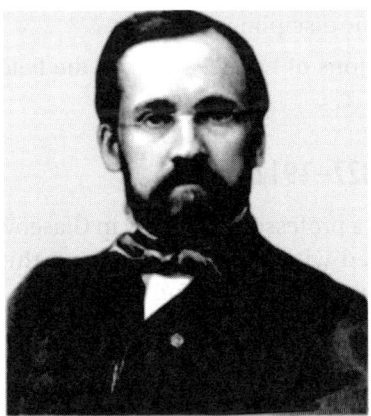

Fig. 1.1: Louis Pasteur.

> **Box 1.1:** Contributions of Louis Pasteur in microbiology.
>
> 1. Coined the term Microbiology.
> 2. **Proposed germ theory of disease:** He established that putrefaction and fermentation was the result of microbial activity.
> 3. **Disapproved theory of spontaneous generation.**
> 4. **Developed sterilization techniques:** He introduced sterilization techniques and developed the steam sterilizer, hot-air oven, and autoclave in the course of these studies.
> 5. **Developed methods and techniques for cultivation of microorganisms**
> 6. Studies on pebrine (silkworm disease), anthrax, chicken cholera, and hydrophobia.
> 7. **Pasteurization:** He devised the process of destroying bacteria, known as pasteurization (1863–65).
> 8. **Coined the term** *vaccine*.
> 9. **Discovery of the process of attenuation and chicken cholera vaccine.**
> 10. **Developed live attenuated anthrax vaccine:** He attenuated cultures of the anthrax bacillus by incubation at high temperature (42–43°C) and proved that inoculation of such cultures in animals induced specific protection against **anthrax**.
> 11. **Developed rabies vaccine:** The crowning achievement of Pasteur was the successful application of the principle of vaccination to the prevention of rabies or hydrophobia, in human beings and developed Pasteur rabies vaccine in 1885.
> 12. **Noticed Pneumococci.**

him to take interest in microorganisms. His discoveries revolutionized medical practice, although he never studied medicine.

Father of Microbiology: He is known as **"Father of Microbiology"** because his contribution led to the development of *Microbiology* as a separate scientific discipline.

The contributions of Louis Pasteur in the field of Microbiology are given in **Box 1.1**.

Joseph Lister (1827–1912)

Joseph Lister was a professor of Surgery in Glasgow Royal Infirmary. He was impressed with Pasteur's study on the involvement of microorganisms in fermentation and putrefaction.

- ❖ **Developed a system of antiseptic surgery:** He developed a system of antiseptic surgery designed to prevent microorganisms from entering wounds. It also provided strong evidence for the role of microorganism in disease because phenol, which killed bacteria, also prevented wound infections.

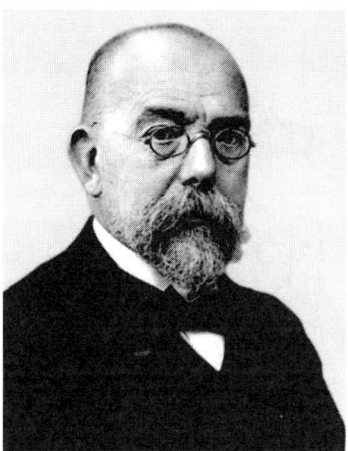

Fig. 1.2: Robert Koch.

- **Father of modern surgery:** He established the guiding principle of antisepsis for good surgical practice and it was milestone in the evolution of surgical practice from the era of "laudable pus" to modern aseptic techniques. For this work he is called the "**Father of Modern Surgery**".

Robert Koch (1843–1910)

Robert Koch was the German physician **(Fig. 1.2)**. The first direct demonstration of the role of bacteria in carrying disease came by the study of anthrax by Koch. Winner of the Nobel Prize in 1905, Robert Koch is known as "**Father of Bacteriology**".

Contributions of Robert Koch

1. **Staining techniques:** He described **methods for the easy microscopic examination of bacteria** in dried, fixed films stained with aniline dyes (1877).
2. **Hanging drop method:** He was the first to use **hanging drop method** by studying bacterial motility.
3. **Methods for isolating pure cultures of bacteria:** He devised a **simple method for isolating pure cultures of bacteria** by plating out mixed material on a solid culture medium and to isolate pure cultures of pathogens.

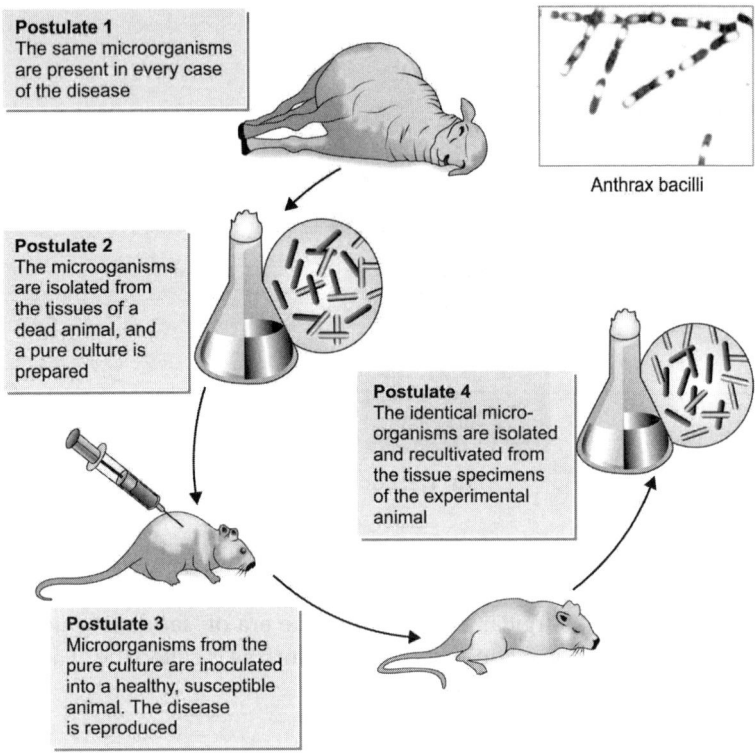

Fig. 1.3: Demonstration of Koch's postulates.

4. **Discoveries** of the **causal agents of anthrax (1876), tuberculosis (1882), and cholera (1883).**
5. **Koch's postulates:** Robert Koch proved that microorganisms cause diseases. Koch used the criteria to establish the relationship between *Bacillus anthracis* and anthrax **(Fig. 1.3)**. His criteria for proving the causal relationship between a microorganism and a specific disease are known as **Koch's postulates (1876)**, which are used today to prove that a particular microorganism causes a particular disease **(Box 1.2)**.
6. **Koch's phenomenon: Robert Koch (1890)** observed that a guinea pig already infected with the bacillus responded with an exaggerated response when injected with the tubercle bacillus or its protein. This hypersensitivity reaction is known as **Koch's phenomenon.**

> **Box 1.2:** Koch's postulates.
>
> Koch's postulates are a series of guidelines for the experimental study of infectious disease. According to these, a microorganism can be accepted as the causative agent of an infectious disease only **(Fig. 1.3)** if the following conditions are satisfied:
> - **Postulate 1:** The organism should be regularly found in the lesions of the disease.
> - **Postulate 2:** It should be possible to isolate the organism in pure culture from the lesions.
> - **Postulate 3:** Inoculation of the pure culture into suitable laboratory animals should reproduce the lesion of the disease.
> - **Postulate 4:** It should be possible to reisolate the organism in pure culture from the lesions produced in the experimental animals.
>
> Subsequently an additional fifth criterion introduced that states the specific antibodies to the organism should be demonstrable in the serum of patients suffering from the disease.
>
> **Limitations of Koch's postulates:** Even today Koch's postulates are considered whenever a new infectious disease arises. These criteria have proved invaluable in identifying pathogens, but they cannot always be met, for example, some organisms (including all viruses) cannot be grown on artificial media, and some are pathogenic only for man. *Mycobacterium leprae*, a causative agent of leprosy, has not been cultured on artificial medium so far and not fulfilling Koch's postulates.

■ DISCOVERY OF VIRUSES

As a science, virology evolved later than bacteriology. Although the physical nature of viruses was not fully revealed until the invention of the electron microscope, the infections they cause have been known and feared since the dawn of history.

Immunity and Immunization

Edward Jenner (1749–1823)

The first scientific attempt at artificial immunizations in the late eighteenth century was taken by **Edward Jenner (1749-1823)** from England. Edward Jenner is known as the "**Father of Immunology**".

■ SEROTHERAPY AND CHEMOTHERAPY

Antisera: The work of **Behring and Kitasato** led to the successful use of antisera raised in animals for the treatment of patients with diphtheria, tetanus, pneumonia and other diseases. Antisera were the only specific therapeutic agents available for the management of infectious diseases till **Domagk (1935)** initiated scientific chemotherapy with the discovery of prontosil.

Magic bullet: Ehrlich (1909) discovered **salvarsan (arsphenamine)**, sometimes called the **"magic bullet"** was capable of destroying the spirochete of syphilis with only moderate toxic effects.

Antibiotics—a "fortunate accident": Sir Alexander Fleming (1881-1955) made accidental discovery that the fungus *Penicillium notatum* produces a substance which destroys staphylococci.

■ BRANCHES OF MICROBIOLOGY

- ❖ **Bacteriology:** The study of bacteria
- ❖ **Mycology:** The study of fungi
- ❖ **Parasitology:** The study of parasites
- ❖ **Immunology:** The study of the immune system
- ❖ **Virology:** The study of viruses

■ SCOPE OF MICROBIOLOGY IN NURSING

1. **To promote health:** Nursing care in the hospital and community is of paramount importance to promote health and it is considered to be the backbone of public health. To attain perfection in this profession, nurses should acquire sound knowledge of nursing microbiology, as nursing is an interdependent profession influenced by the recent scientific and technological advances of nursing sciences. Microbiology is needed in nursing to take care of patient and to protect oneself from pathogenic microorganisms.

    Aseptic technique becomes almost second nature to the nurse, who practices it daily. However, the patient is less aware of the factors that promote the spread of infection or of the ways to prevent its transmission. A nurse will be obliged to educate patients about the nature of infection and the techniques to use in planning or controlling its spread.

2. **Diagnosis and treatment of infection:** The role of the laboratory in assisting clinicians in the diagnosis of infection is to provide the physician with information concerning the presence or absence of microorganisms that may be involved in the infectious disease process. These individuals and facilities also determine the susceptibility of microorganisms to antimicrobial agents.

Application of knowledge of medical microbiology at the bedside of patients during nursing care will be possible due to nursing microbiology and nurses should acquire sound knowledge of nursing microbiology.

3. **Sterilization and disinfection:** Pathogenic microorganisms are infectious agents. Unwashed hands, wound dressings, soiled linen, and decaying teeth provide ideal areas for pathogenic growth. The strength of the microorganism, the number of microorganisms present, the effectiveness of a person's immune system, and the length of exposure to the microorganisms determine a pathogen's ability to produce disease. A nurse has a duty to provide a safe environment for a patient which can be accomplished by performing hand hygiene, donning gloves, **disinfection** (the use of a chemical that can be applied to objects to destroy microorganisms), using an **antiseptic** (a substance that tends to inhibit the growth and reproduction of microorganisms—may be used on humans), and sterilization.

4. **Prophylaxis (to prevent the spread of infection): Nurses** should have knowledge about the mode of spread of infection. In the final analysis the patient's well-being and health can benefit significantly from information provided by the clinical microbiology laboratory. Clinical microbiologists and clinical microbiology laboratories perform many services, all related to the identification and control of pathogens.

5. **Diagnosis and control of hospital infection (infection control team):** An infection control team of workers, headed by the **infection control doctor**. The *infection control nurse* is the key member of this team. The functions of this team include **surveillance and control of infection and monitoring of hygiene practices,** advising the infection control committee on matters of policy relating to the prevention of infection and the education of all staff in the microbiologically safe performance of procedures.

Many agencies employ nurses who are especially trained in infection prevention and control. They are responsible for advising hospital personnel on the development and implementation of safe patient care delivery practices and for monitoring infection outbreaks within the healthcare agency.

NOBEL PRIZES AWARDED FOR RESEARCH IN MICROBIOLOGY

The number of Nobel laureates in Medicine and Physiology for their contribution in microbiology is evidence of the positive contribution made to human health by the science of microbiology. About one-third of these have been awarded to scientists working on microbiological problems (**Table 1.1**).

TABLE 1.1: Nobel laureates for research in microbiology.

Year	Nobel laureates	Contribution
1901	Emil A von Behring	Developed a diphtheria antitoxin
1902	Ronald Ross	Discovered how malaria is transmitted
1905	Robert Koch	Tuberculosis—discovery of causative agent
1907	CLA Laveron	Discovery of malaria parasite in an unstained preparation of fresh blood
1908	Paul Ehrlich and Elie Metchnikoff	Developed theories on immunity. Described phagocytosis, the intake of solid materials by cells
1913	Charles Richet	Anaphylaxis
1919	Jules Bordet	Discovered roles of complement and antibody in cytolysis, developed complement fixation test
1928	Charles Nicolle	Typhus exanthematicus
1930	Karl Landsteiner	Described ABO blood groups; solidified chemical basis for antigen-antibody reactions
1939	Gerhardt Domagk	Antibacterial effect of prontosil
1945	Alexander Fleming, Ernst Chain, and Howard Florey	Discovered penicillin
1951	Max Theiler	Yellow fever vaccine
1952	Selman A Waksman	Development of streptomycin. He coined the term "antibiotic"
1954	John F Enders, Thomas H Weller, and Frederick C Robbins	Cultured poliovirus in cell cultures
1960	Sir Macfarlane Burnet and Sir Peter Brian Medawar	Immunological tolerance, clonal selection theory
1962	James D Watson, Francis H C Crick, and Maurice AF Wilkins	Double helix structure of deoxyribonucleic acid (DNA)

Contd...

Contd...

Year	Nobel laureates	Contribution
1966	Francois Jacob, Andre Lwoff and Jacques Monod	Regulatory mechanisms in microbial genes (concept of "lac operon")
1966	Peyton Rous	Viral oncogenes (avian sarcoma)
1968	Robert Holley, Har Gobind Khorana, and Marshall W Nirenberg	Genetic code
1969	Max Delbruck, AD Hershey and Salvador Luria	Mechanism of virus infection in living cells
1972	Gerald M Edelman and Rodney R Porter	Described the nature and structure of antibodies
1975	David Baltimore, Renata Dulbecco and Howard M Temin	Interactions between tumor viruses and genetic material of the cells
1977	Rosalyn Yalow	Developed immunoassay
1980	Baruj Benacerraf, Jean Dausset and George Snell	HLA antigens
1984	Cesar Milstein, Georges Kohler, Niels K Jerne	Developed hybridoma technology for production of monoclonal antibodies
1987	S Tonegawa	Described the genetics of antibody production
1989	J Michael Bishop and Harold E Varmus	Discovered cancer-causing genes called oncogenes
1990	Joseph E Murray and E Donnall Thomas	Performed the first successful organ transplants by using immunosuppressive agents
1993	Kary B Mullis	Discovered the polymerase chain reaction (PCR) to amplify DNA
1996	Peter C Doherty and Rolf M Zinkernagel	Cell-mediated immune defenses
1997	Stanley B Prusiner	Prion discovery
2001	Leland H Hartwell, Paul M Nurse, and R Timothy Hunt	Discovered genes that encode proteins regulating cell division
2005	Barry J Marshall and J Robin Warren	*Helicobacter pylori* and its role in gastritis and peptic ulcer disease
2007	Mario R Capecchi, Oliver Smithies and Sir Martin J Evans	Creation of knockout mice for stem cell research
2008	Luc Montagnier and Francoise Barre-Sinoussi	Discovery of human immunodeficiency virus
	Harald zur Hausen	Human papillomaviruses causing cervical cancer

Contd...

Contd...

Year	Nobel laureates	Contribution
2011	Bruce A Beutler and Jules A Hoffmann	Discoveries concerning the activation of innate immunity
	Ralph M Steinman	Discovery of dendritic cell and its role in adaptive immunity
2012	Sir John B Gurdon and S Yamanaka	Discovery that mature cells can be programmed to become pluripotent
2015	William C Campbell and Satoshi Omura	For the discovery concerning a novel therapy against infections caused by roundworm parasites
		For the discovery concerning a novel therapy against malaria
2018	James P Allison and Tasuku Honjo	For the discovery of cancer by inhibition of negative immune regulation
2020	Harvey J Alter, Michael Houghton and Charles M Rice	Discovery of hepatitis C virus

KEY POINTS

- ❖ Microbiology is the study of living organisms of microscopic size.
- ❖ Antony van Leeuwenhoek was the first person to describe microorganisms.
- ❖ **Louis Pasteur** is known as **"Father of Microbiology".**
- ❖ **Robert Koch:**
  - Koch developed the techniques required to grow bacteria on solid media and to isolate pure cultures of pathogens.
  - Koch's postulates are used to prove a direct relationship between a suspected pathogen and a disease.

IMPORTANT QUESTIONS

1. Write short notes on:
   a. Contributions of Louis Pasteur
   b. Contributions of Robert Koch
   c. Koch's postulates
2. Write briefly on scope of microbiology in nursing.

Chapter 1: Historical Development of Microbiology

MULTIPLE CHOICE QUESTIONS

1. Who was the first person to describe microorganisms?
   a. Louis Pasteur
   b. Robert Koch
   c. Paul Ehrlich
   d. Antony van Leeuwenhoek
2. Who is Father of Microbiology?
   a. Louis Pasteur
   b. Robert Koch
   c. Paul Ehrlich
   d. Joseph Lister
3. Who is Father of Bacteriology?
   a. Louis Pasteur
   b. Robert Koch
   c. Paul Ehrlich
   d. Joseph Lister
4. Who is Father of Immunology?
   a. Louis Pasteur
   b. Robert Koch
   c. Paul Ehrlich
   d. Edward Jenner

ANSWERS
1. d   2. a   3. b   4. d

SECTION 2

Microorganisms

Section Outline

- ❖ Morphology of Bacteria
- ❖ Physiology of Bacteria
- ❖ Normal Microbial Flora of the Human Body
- ❖ Pathogenesis and Common Diseases
- ❖ Methods for Study of Microbes
- ❖ Culture Media and Culture Methods

CHAPTER 2

Morphology of Bacteria

Learning Objectives

After reading and studying this chapter, you should be able to:
- Differentiate between prokaryotes and eukaryotes.
- Describe anatomy of bacterial cell.
- Describe cell envelope.
- Describe bacterial cell wall.
- Discuss capsule or bacterial capsule.
- Describe bacterial flagellae.
- Describe fimbriae or pili.
- Discuss bacterial spores or endospores.
- Explain L-forms of bacteria.

■ INTRODUCTION

Microorganisms are generally regarded as living forms that are microscopic in size and relatively simple, usually unicellular in structure. The bacteria are single-celled organisms that reproduce by simple division, i.e., binary fission.

■ NAMING AND CLASSIFYING MICROORGANISMS

Microorganisms are a heterogeneous group of several distinct classes of living beings. Whittaker's system recognizes five-kingdoms of living things—**Monera (bacteria), Protista, Fungi, Plantae, and Animalia**. Five kingdoms have been modified further by the development of **three domains, or Superkingdoms** system—the **Bacteria,** the **Archaea** (meaning ancient), and the **Eukarya**.

Nomenclature

The system of nomenclature (naming) for organisms in use today was established in 1735 by Carolus Linnaeus. Scientific names are Latinized. Scientific nomenclature assigns each organism two names—the genus (plural: genera) is the first name and is always capitalized; the specific epithet (species name) follows and is not capitalized. The organism is referred to by both the genus and the specific epithet, and both names are underlined or italicized. With the initial of the genus followed by the specific epithet, e.g., *Staphylococcus aureus* (*Staphylococcus*—Genus; *aureus*—Species).

Comparison of Prokaryotic Cells Eukaryotic Cells

All living organisms on earth are composed of one or the other of two types of cells ***prokaryotic*** cells and ***eukaryotic*** cells (**Table 2.1**).
1. **Prokaryotes:—Bacteria and Archaea:** All bacteria and blue-green algae are prokaryotes.
2. **Eukaryotes—Eukarya:** Other algae (excluding blue-green algae), fungi, slime molds, protozoa, higher plants, and animals are eukaryotic **(Table 2.1)**.

TABLE 2.1: Principle differences between prokaryotic and eukaryotic cells.

Characteristic	Prokaryotic	Eukaryotic
Size (approximate)	0.5–3 μm	>5 μm
Nucleus		
Nuclear membrane	Absent	Present
Nucleolus	Absent	Present
Chromosome	One (circular)	More than one (linear)
Deoxyribonucleoprotein	Absent	Present
Division	By binary fission	By mitosis
Cytoplasm		
Cytoplasmic streaming	Absent	Present
Mitochondria	Absent	Present
Golgi apparatus	Absent	Present
Lysosomes	Absent	Present
Pinocytosis	Absent	Present
Endoplasmic reticulum	Absent	Present
Chemical composition		
Sterol	Absent	Present
Muramic acid	Present	Absent
Examples	Eubacteria, archaea All bacteria and blue-green algae	Fungi, slime moulds, protozoa, higher plants, and animals including humans

Size of Bacteria

The unit of measurement in bacteriology is the micron (µ) or micrometer (µm):
 1 µ or µm = a millionth part of a meter or a thousandth of a millimeter.
 1 millimicron (mµ) or nanometer (nm) = one thousandth of a micron or one millionth of a millimeter.
 1 Angstrom unit (A) = one tenth of a nanometer.
 The diameter of the smallest body that can be resolved and seen clearly with naked eye is 200 µm. Bacteria of medical importance generally measure 0.2–1.5 µm in diameter and about 3–5 µm in length. To see bacteria a light microscope must be used.

■ STUDY OF BACTERIA

Stained Preparations

Because most microorganisms appear almost colorless when viewed through a standard light microscope, we often must prepare them for observation. Staining simply means coloring the microorganisms with a dye that emphasizes certain structures.

Routine methods for staining of bacteria involve drying and fixing smears, procedures that kill them. Fixing simultaneously kills the microorganisms and attaches them to the slide. It also preserves various parts of microbes in their natural state with only minimal distortion. Various staining techniques are commonly used in bacteriology (**See Chapter 20: Identification of common microbes under the microscope**).

Shape of Bacteria

Depending on their shape, bacteria are classified into several varieties (**Fig. 2.1**):
1. **Cocci:** Cocci (from *kokkos* meaning berry) are spherical, or nearly spherical.
2. **Bacilli:** Bacilli (from *baculus* meaning rod) are relatively straight, rod shaped (cylindrical) cells. In some of the bacilli the length of the cells may be equal to width. Such bacillary forms are known as coccobacilli and have to be carefully differentiated from cocci.

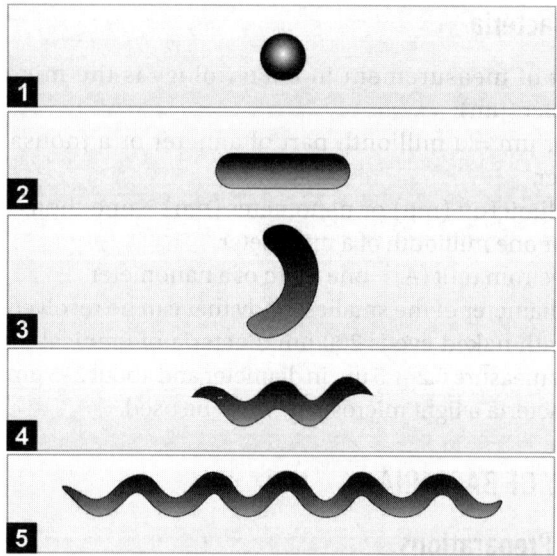

Fig. 2.1: Shapes of bacteria: 1. Coccus; 2. Bacillus; 3. Vibrio; 4. Spirillum; 5. Spirochete.

3. **Vibrios:** Vibrios are curved or comma-shaped rods.
4. **Spirilla**: Spirilla are rigid spiral or helical forms.
5. **Spirochetes**: Spirochetes (from speira meaning coil and chaite meaning hair) are flexuous spiral forms.
6. **Mycoplasmas**: These are cell wall-deficient bacteria and hence do not possess a stable morphology.

Arrangement of Bacterial Cells

Pathogenic bacterial species appear as sphere (cocci), rods (bacilli), and spirals. Bacteria sometimes show characteristic cellular arrangement or grouping **(Figs. 2.2A and B)**. The type of cellular arrangement is determined by the plane through which binary fission takes place and by the tendency of the daughter cells to remain attached even after division.

Cocci Arrangement

i. **Diplococci:** Cocci may be arranged in pairs (diplococci) when cocci divide and remain together.

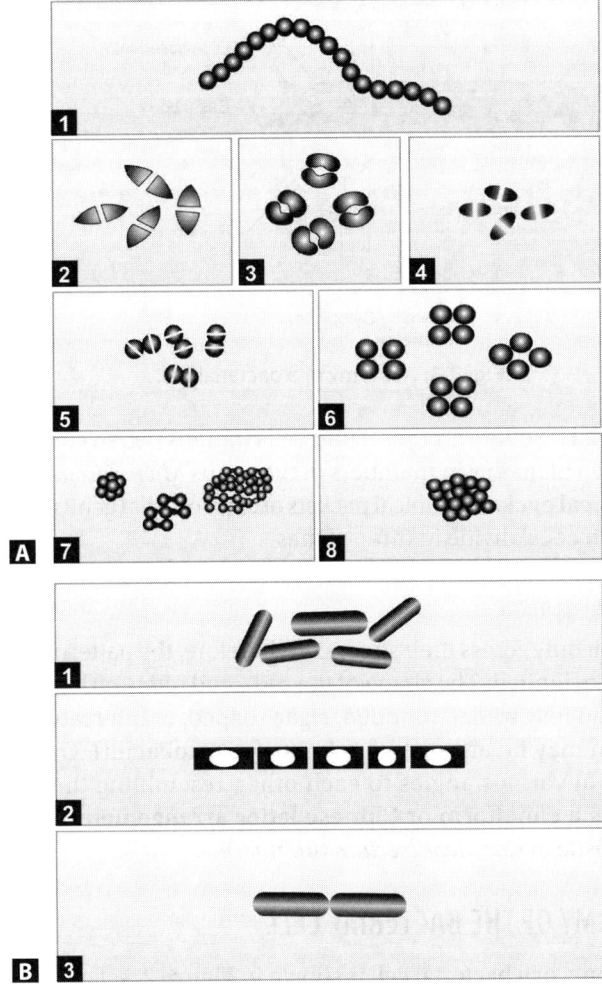

Figs. 2.2A and B: Arrangement of bacteria: (A) Cocci: 1. Streptococci, 2. Pneumococci, 3. Gonococci, 4. Meningococci, 5. *Neisseria catarrhalis*, 6. *Gaffkya tetragena*, 7. Sarcina, 8. Staphylococci; (B) Bacilli: 1. Bacilli in cluster, 2. Bacilli in chains (*B. anthrax*), 3. Diplobacilli (*K. pneumoniae*).

ii. **Long chains:** Long chains (*Streptococcus, Enterococcus*, and *Lactococcus*) when cells adhere after repeated divisions in one plane.
iii. **Grape-like clusters:** Grape-like clusters (staphylococci) when cocci divide in random planes.

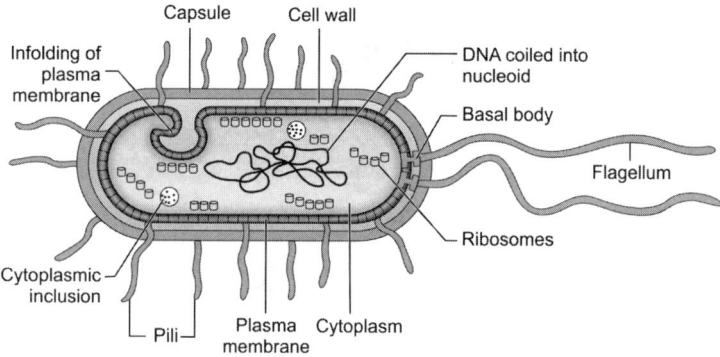

Fig. 2.3: Anatomy of a bacterial cell.

    iv. **Tetrads:** Square groups of four cells (tetrads) when cocci divide in two planes as in members of the genus *Micrococcus*.
    v. **Cubical packets:** Cubical packets of eight of cells (genus *Sarcina*) when cocci divide in three planes.

Bacilli Arrangement

Bacilli split only across their short axis, therefore, the patterns formed by them are limited. The shape of the rod's end often varies between species and may be flat, rounded, cigar-shaped, or bifurcated. Some bacilli too may be arranged in **chains** (streptobacilli). Others are arranged at various angles to each other, resembling the letter V presenting a **cuneiform** or **Chinese letter arrangement** and it is a characteristic of *Corynebacterium diphtheriae*.

■ ANATOMY OF THE BACTERIAL CELL

The anatomy of a bacterial cell is shown in **Figure 2.3**. The chemical structures of the bacterial cell wall are shown in **Figure 2.4**.

Bacterial Cell Components

It can be divided into:
A. Cell envelope and its appendages.
    a. **The outer layer or cell envelope** consists of two components:
       1. **Cell wall**
       2. **Cytoplasmic or plasma membrane**—beneath cell wall
    b. Cellular appendages—capsule, fimbriae, and flagella

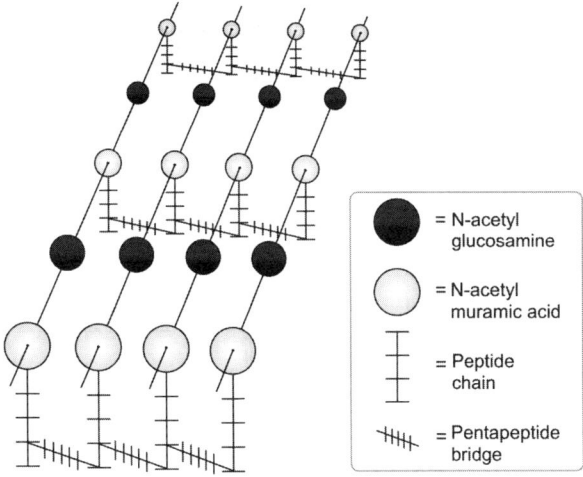

Fig. 2.4: Chemical structure of bacterial cell wall.

B. **Cell interior:** Those structures and substances that are bounded by the cytoplasmic membrane compose the cell interior and include **cytoplasm, cytoplasmic inclusions (mesosomes, ribosomes, inclusion granules, vacuoles) and a single circular chromosome of deoxyribonucleic acid (DNA).**

Cell Envelope and its Appendages

The Outer Layer or Cell Envelope

1. *Cell wall:* The cell wall is the layer that lies just outside the plasma membrane. It is thick, strong, and relatively rigid.
   Gram-positive bacterial cell wall: In gram-positive bacteria, the cell wall consists mainly of peptidoglycan and teichoic acids (**Fig. 2.5**).
   a. **Peptidoglycan**: It is thicker and stronger than those of gram-negative bacteria.
   b. **Teichoic acid:** In addition, the cell walls of gram-positive bacteria contain *teichoic acids.*
   Gram-negative cell wall: The gram-negative cell wall is structurally quite different from that of gram-positive cells (**Fig. 2.6**). It consists of **peptidoglycan and lipoprotein, outer membrane, and lipopolysaccharide.**
   a. **Peptidoglycan layer**: It is bonded to lipoproteins covalently in the outer membrane and plasma membrane and is in the

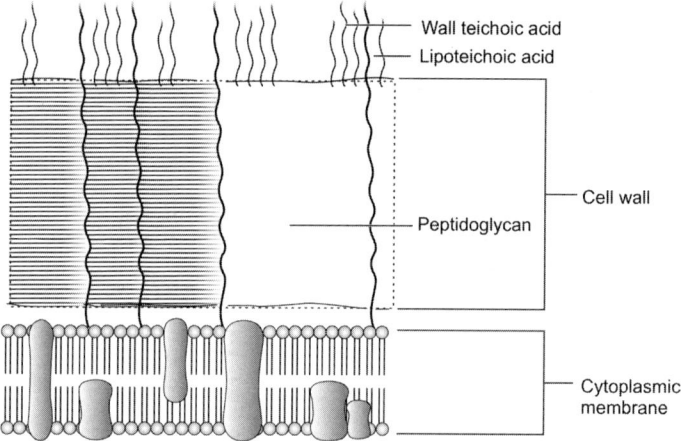

Fig. 2.5: Gram-positive cell wall.

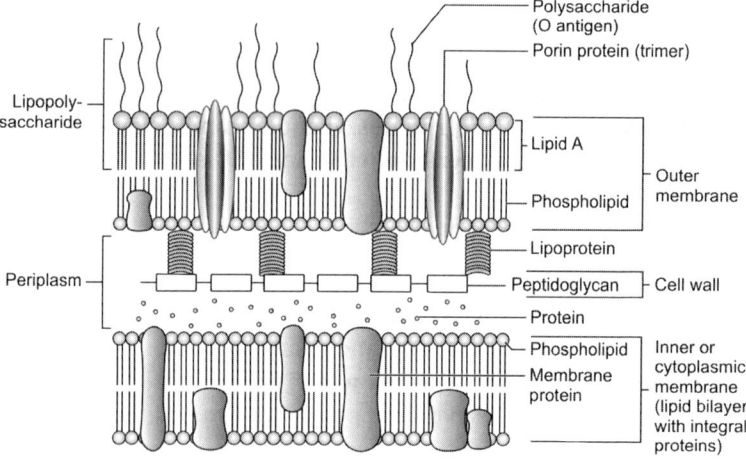

Fig. 2.6: Gram-negative cell wall.

periplasmic, a gel-like fluid between the outer membrane and plasma membrane.

b. **Lipoproteins:** Lipoproteins or murein lipoproteins attach to the peptidoglycan, and to the outer membrane.

c. **Outer membrane:** External to the peptidoglycan and attached to it by lipoprotein is the outer membrane. It is bilayered structure. Its inner leaflet is composed of phospholipid and outer leaflet by lipopolysaccharide (LPS).

TABLE 2.2: Comparison of cell walls of gram-positive and gram-negative bacteria.

Characteristic	Gram-positive	Gram-negative
Thickness	Thicker	Thinner
Peptidoglycan	Thick layer (16–80 nm)	Thin layer (2 nm)
Teichoic acid	Present	Absent
Variety of amino acids	Few	Several
Aromatic and sulfur containing amino acids	Absent or scant	Present
Lipids	Absent or scant	Present
Porin proteins	Absent	Present
Periplasmic region	Absent	Present

    d. **Lipopolysaccharide:** LPS consists of three components:
       i. **Lipid A** is the lipid portion of LPS and is embedded in the top layer of the outer membrane. Lipid A functions as an **endotoxin**. All the toxicity of the endotoxin is due to lipid A, i.e., pyrogenicity, lethal effect, tissue necrosis, etc.
      ii. **The core polysaccharide** is attached to lipid A.
      iii. **O polysaccharide**: It is known as **O antigen**. Differences between cell wall of gram-positive and gram-negative bacteria are shown in **Table 2.2**.
2. *Cytoplasmic (plasma) membrane (Table 2.2)*
   Structure: It is thin (5–10 nm thick), elastic and can only be seen with electron microscope.

   Functions of cytoplasmic membrane:
     i. **Semipermeable membrane**
     ii. **Housing enzymes and proteins**
     iii. **Generation of chemical energy**
     iv. **Cell motility**
     v. **Mediation of chromosomal segregation during replication**

Cellular Appendages

Capsule or Slime Layer

Structure: Many bacteria synthesize large amount of extracellular polymer in their natural environments. When the polymer forms a condensed, well-defined layer closely surrounding the cell, it is called the capsule as in the pneumococcus. If the polymer is easily washed off and does not appear to be associated with the cell in any definite fashion, it is referred as a slime layer.

Composition of capsules and slime layers: Capsules and slime layers usually are composed of polysaccharide (e.g., *Pneumococcus*) or of polypeptide in some bacteria (e.g., *Bacillus anthracis* and *Yersinia pestis*).

Capsulated bacteria: *Streptococcus pneumoniae*, several groups of streptococci, *Neisseria meningitidis*, *Klebsiella*, *Haemophilus influenzae*, *Yersinia* and *Bacillus*.

Demonstration of Capsule

i. **Gram stain:** Slime has little affinity for basic dyes and is not visible in Gram-stained smears.
ii. **Special capsule staining techniques**: Usually, employing copper salts as mordants.
iii. **India ink staining (negative staining):** The capsule appears as a clear halo around the bacterium, against a dark background in the film **(Fig. 2.7)**.
iv. **Electron microscope**
v. **Serological methods:** When a suspension of a capsulated bacterium is mixed with its specific anticapsular serum and

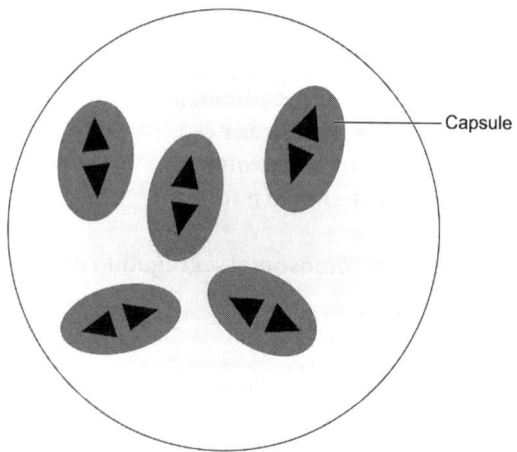

Fig. 2.7: Pneumococci negatively stained with India ink to show capsule.

examined under the microscope, the capsule becomes very prominent and appears "swollen" due to an increase in its refractivity. It is known as the **capsule-swelling reaction** or **Quellung reaction** (Quellung-*Ger; swelling*), described by Neufeld (1902).

Functions of Capsule
i. **Virulence factor—by inhibiting phagocytosis**
ii. **Protection of the cell wall**
iii. **Identification and typing of bacteria**

Flagella

Motile bacteria possess one or more unbranched, long, sinuous filaments called **flagella**, which are the organs of locomotion.

Structure (Fig. 2.7): They are 3–20 μm long with uniform diameter (0.01–0.013 μm) and terminate in a square tip. Flagella consists of largely or entirely of a protein, **flagellin**.

Parts and Composition
Each flagellum consists of three parts:
1. Filament
2. Hook
3. Basal body

Arrangement/Types (Figs. 2.8 and 2.9)
These are four types of flagella arrangement:
1. **Monotrichous**—single polar flagellum, e.g., *Vibrio cholera*.
2. **Amphitrichous**—single flagellum at both ends, e.g., *Alcaligenes faecalis*.
3. **Lophotrichous**—tuft of flagella at one or both ends, e.g., spirilla.
4. **Peritrichous**—flagella surrounding the cell, e.g., typhoid bacilli.

Demonstration of Flagella
Flagella are about 0.02 μm in thickness and hence beyond the resolution limit of the light microscope. The following methods are used for its demonstration:
i. **Dark ground illumination**
ii. **Special staining methods**: In which their thickness is increased by mordanting

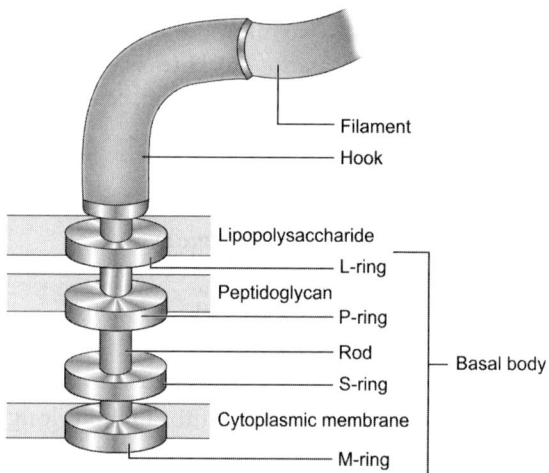

Fig. 2.8: The structure of bacterial flagellum.

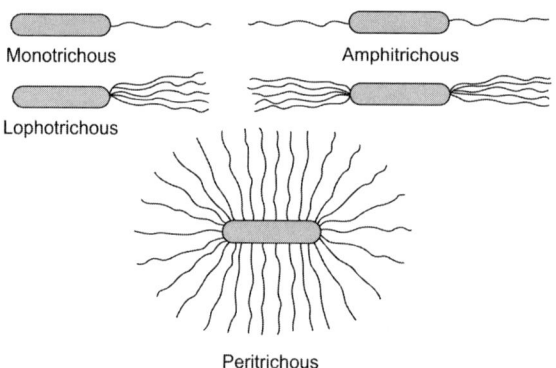

Fig. 2.9: Arrangement of flagella.

iii. **Electron microscopy**
iv. **Indirect methods**: Indirect methods by which motility of bacteria can be seen or demonstrated.
    a. Microscopically in fluid suspensions (in a hanging drop or under a coverslip)
    b. **By spread of bacterial growth as a film over agar,** e.g., swarming growth of *Proteus* spp.
    c. **Turbidity spreading through semisolid agar,** e.g., Craigie tube method.

Fimbria or Pili

Structure and synthesis: Many gram-negative bacteria have short, fine, hair-like surface appendages which are called **fimbriae or pili**. They are shorter and thinner than flagella (0.1–1.5 μm in length and uniform width between 4 and 8 nm) and emerge from the cell wall. They originate in the **cytoplasmic membrane** and are composed of protein termed **pilins** like flagella.

Demonstration of Fimbriae
1. Electron microscopy
2. Hemagglutination

Functions of Pilli
Two classes can be distinguished on the basis of their function: (1) **Ordinary (common) pili** and (2) **sex pili**.

Cell Interior

1. **Cytoplasm:** The cytoplasm of the bacterial cell is a viscous watery solution or soft gel, containing a variety of organic or inorganic solutes, and numerous ribosomes and polysomes.
2. **Ribosomes:** The ribosomes are the location for all bacterial protein synthesis.
3. **Mesosomes (chondrioids)**
   Structure: These are convoluted or multilaminated membranous bodies formed as invaginations of the plasma membrane into the cytoplasm.
   Functions of mesosomes:
   i. Compartmenting of deoxyribonucleic acid (DNA)
   ii. Sites of the respiratory enzymes
4. **Intracytoplasmic inclusions:** These bodies are usually for storage. They consist of **volutin (polyphosphate), lipid, glycogen, starch or sulfur.**
5. **Bacterial nucleus:**
   Structure: The genetic material of a bacterial cell is contained in a single, long molecule of double-stranded DNA which can be extracted in the form of a closed circular thread about 1 mm (1,000 μm) long, about 1,000 times the length of the cell. The bacterial chromosome is haploid and replicates by simple fission. Bacterial nucleus does not possess nuclear membrane.

Plasmids: Bacteria may possess extranuclear genetic elements in the cytoplasm consisting of DNA termed *plasmids* or *episomes*.

Function of plasmids: Plasmids are not essential for host growth and reproduction they inhabit, but may **confer on it certain properties**, such as drug resistance, enhanced pathogenicity, which may constitute a survival advantage.

6. **Bacterial spore:** A number of gram-positive bacteria, such as those of the genera *Clostridium* and *Bacillus* can form a special resistant dormant structure called an **endospore** or, simply, **spores**. Endospore develops when essential nutrients are depleted. Sporulation in bacteria, therefore, is not a method of reproduction but of preservation **(Figs. 2.10 and 2.11)**.

Sporulation: Spore formation, sporogenesis or sporulation normally commences when growth ceases due to lack of nutrients, depletion of the nitrogen or carbon source (or both) being the most significant factor.

Stages: It is a complex process and may be divided into several stages.

Spore septum:

Forespore: The spore septum becomes a **double-layered membrane** that surrounds the chromosome and cytoplasm. Structure, entirely enclosed within the original cell, is called a **forespore.**

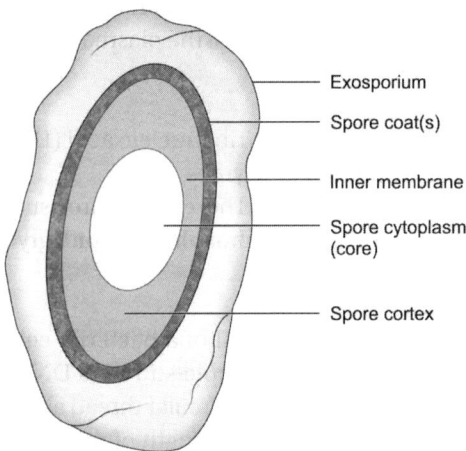

Fig. 2.10: Bacterial spore (cross-section).

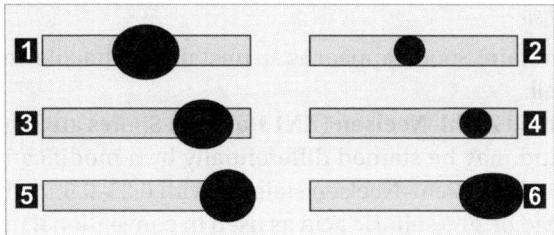

Fig. 2.11: Types of spores: 1. Central, bulging, 2. Central, not bulging, 3. Subterminal, bulging, 4. Subterminal, not bulging, 5. Terminal, spherical, 6. Terminal, oval.

Spore coat: The forespore is subsequently completely encircled by dividing septum as a double layered membrane. The two spore membranes now engage in active synthesis of various layers of the spore. The inner layer becomes the **inner membrane**. Between the two layers there is laid **spore cortex** and outer layer is transformed into **spore coat** which consists of several layers. In some species from outer layer also develops **exosporium** which bears ridges and folds **(Fig. 2.10)**.

Germination: Germination is the process of conversion of a spore into vegetative cells under suitable conditions.

Shape and Position of Spores

Spores may be central (equatorial), subterminal (close to one end), or terminal **(Fig. 2.10)**. The appearance may be spherical, ovoid or elongated, and being narrower that the cell, or broader and bulging it. The diameter of spore may be same or less than the width of bacteria (Bacillus), or may be wider than the bacillary body producing a distension or bulge in the cell (*Clostridium*).

Resistance

Bacterial spores constitute some of the most resistant forms of life. Spores of all medically important species are destroyed by autoclaving at 120°C for 15 minutes. Methods of sterilization and disinfection should ensure that spores also are destroyed. Sporulation helps bacteria survive for long periods under unfavorable environments.

Demonstration

i. **Gram stain:** Spores appear as an unstained refractile body within the cell.
ii. **Modified Ziehl-Neelsen (ZN) staining:** Spores are slightly acid-fast and may be stained differentially by a modification of the ZN method. Ziehl-Neelsen staining with 0.25–0.5% sulfuric acid (instead of 20% sulfuric acid as used in conventional method) as decoloring agent is used for spore staining.

Uses of Spores

1. **Importance in food, industrial, and medical microbiology**
2. **Sterilization control:** For proper sterilization, spores of certain species of bacteria are employed as indicator, e.g., *Bacillus stearothermophilus* which is destroyed at a temperature of 121°C for 10–20 minutes (same temperature and time as used in autoclaving). Prior to its use, these spores may be kept in autoclave. Proper sterilization is indicated by the absence of the spores after autoclaving.
3. **Research**

L-Forms of Bacteria (Cell Wall Defective Organisms)

Abnormal forms of the bacteria were named **L-forms** after the Lister Institute, London (hence, the "L").

Colonies of L-phase organisms on agar media are small and have a characteristic **"fried egg"** appearance.

L-forms are **nonpathogenic to laboratory animals.**

KEY POINTS

Microscopy: A simple microscope consists of one lens; a compound microscope has multiple lenses.

Anatomy of bacterial cell

A. Cell envelope and its appendages
B. Cell interior

Endospores are a dormant stage for survival during adverse environmental conditions.

Chapter 2: Morphology of Bacteria

IMPORTANT QUESTIONS

1. Describe briefly the anatomy of bacterial cell.
2. Draw a labeled diagram of bacterial cell. Write briefly on cell wall of bacteria.
3. Write short notes on:
   a. Bacterial cell wall
   b. Capsule or bacterial capsule
   c. Bacterial flagella
   d. Bacterial spores or endospores

MULTIPLE CHOICE QUESTIONS (MCQs)

1. Which of the following is not a distinguishing characteristic of prokaryotic cells?
   a. They usually have a single, circular chromosome
   b. They lack membrane enclosed organelles
   c. They have cell walls containing peptidoglycan
   d. They lack a plasma membrane
2. Peptidoglycan layer of cell wall is thicker in:
   a. Gram-positive bacteria
   b. Gram-negative bacteria
   c. Fungi
   d. Parasites
3. All the following statements are true for lipopolysaccharide, *except*:
   a. It consists of three components: Lipid A, core polysaccharide and O polysaccharide.
   b. Lipid A functions as an endotoxin
   c. It is an integral part of the cell wall of the gram-positive bacteria
   d. Polysaccharide represents a major surface antigen of the bacterial cell
4. A tuft of flagella present at one or both ends of bacterial cell is known as:
   a. Monotrichous
   b. Amphitrichous
   c. Lophotrichous
   d. Peritrichous
5. Which of the following is not true about fimbriae?
   a. They originate in the cytoplasmic membrane.
   b. They are composed of protein.
   c. They may be used for attachment.
   d. They may be used for motility.
6. Which one of the following bacteria is cell wall deficient?
   a. *Escherichia coli*
   b. *Streptococcus aureus*
   c. *Mycoplasma*
   d. *Treponema pallidum*

Section 2: Microorganisms

7. All of the following are spore forming bacteria, *except*:
   a. *Clostridium botulinum*
   b. *Bacillus anthracis*
   c. *Bacillus subtilis*
   d. *Vibrio cholerae*

ANSWERS					
1. d	2. a	3. c	4. c	5. d	6. c
7. d					

CHAPTER 3

Physiology of Bacteria

Learning Objectives

After reading and studying this chapter, you should be able to:
- Explain generation time of bacteria.
- Describe and draw bacterial growth curve.
- Define the atmospheric requirement of microaerophilic bacteria and capnophilic bacteria.

■ PRINCIPLES OF BACTERIAL GROWTH

Bacterial Division

Bacteria divide by **binary fission** where individual cells enlarge and divide to yield two progeny of approximately equal size. Nuclear division precedes cell division. The cell division occurs by a constrictive or pinching process or by the ingrowth of a transverse septum across the cell. The daughter cells may remain partially attached after division in some species.

Generation Time or Doubling Time

The interval of time between two cell divisions, or the time required for a bacterium to give rise to two daughter cells under optimum conditions, is known as the **generation time or doubling time**. **Examples:** In coliform bacilli and many other medically important bacteria, it is about 20 minutes, in tubercle bacilli, it is about 20 hours, and in lepra bacilli, it is about 20 days.

Colonies: Bacteria growing on solid media form **colonies**.

Bacterial Count

Bacteria in a culture medium or clinical specimen can be counted by two methods:
1. **Total count:** This is total number of bacteria present in a specimen irrespective of whether they are living or dead.
2. **Viable count:** This measures only viable (living) cells.

Bacterial Growth Curve

If a suitable liquid medium is inoculated with bacterium and incubated, its growth follows a definitive course. Small samples are taken at regular intervals after inoculation and plotted in relation to time. A plotting of the data will yield a characteristic growth curve (**Fig. 3.1**).

Phases of Bacterial Growth Curve

The bacterial growth curve can be divided into four major phases: Lag phase, exponential or log (logarithmic) phase, stationary phase, and decline phase.
1. **Lag phase:** When microorganisms are introduced into fresh culture medium, usually no immediate increase in cell number

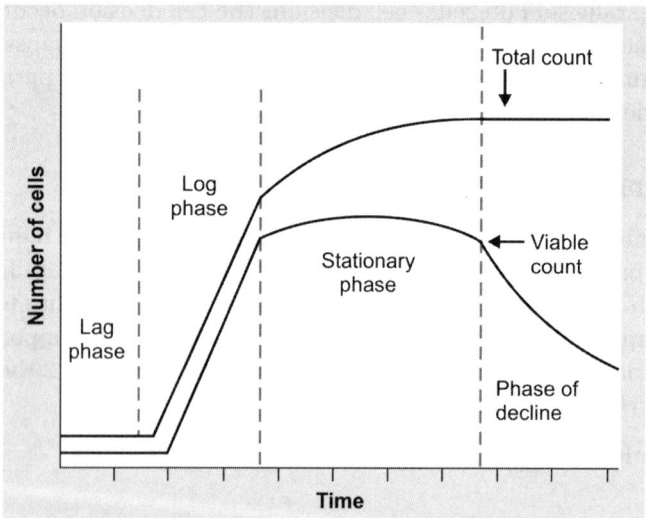

Fig. 3.1: Bacterial growth curve. The viable count shows lag, log, stationary and decline phases. In the total count, the phase of decline is not evident.

occurs, and therefore, this period is called the **lag phase.** After inoculation, there is an increase in cell size at a time when little are no cell division is occurring. This initial period is the time required for adaptation to the new environment, during which the necessary enzymes and metabolic intermediates are built up in adequate quantities for multiplication to proceed.

2. **Log (logarithmic) or exponential phase:** Following the lag phase, the cells start dividing and their numbers increase exponentially or by geometric progression with time. If the logarithm of the viable count is plotted against time, a straight line will be obtained.
3. **Stationary phase:** After a varying period of exponential growth, cell division stops due to depletion of nutrients and accumulation of toxic products. Eventually, growth slows down, and the total bacterial cell number reaches a maximum and stabilizes. The number of progeny cells formed is just enough to replace the number of cells that die. The growth curve becomes horizontal. The viable count remains stationary as equilibrium exists between the dying cells and the newly formed cells.
4. **Decline or death phase:** The death phase is the period when the population decreases due to cell death. Eventually, the rate of death exceeds the rate of reproduction, and the number of viable cells declines. Like bacterial growth, death is exponential. Cell death may also be caused by autolysis besides nutrient deprivation and buildup of toxic wastes. Finally, after a variable period, all the cells die and culture becomes sterile.

Bacterial Nutrition

The minimum nutritional requirements for growth and multiplication of bacteria are water, a source of carbon, a source of nitrogen, and some inorganic salts. The water content of bacterial cells can vary from 75 to 90% of the total weight and is the vehicle for the entry of all cells and for the elimination of all waste products. It participates in the metabolic reactions and also forms an integral part of the protoplasm.

Categories of Requirements

The requirements for microbial growth can be divided into two main categories: Chemical and physical.

A. **Chemical requirements:** Chemical requirements include sources of carbon, nitrogen, sulfur, phosphorus, trace elements, oxygen, and organic growth factors.

B. **Physical requirements:** Physical factors influence microbial growth.

Factors Influencing Microbial Growth

1. Temperature

Optimum temperature: The temperature at which growth occur best is known as the "**optimum temperature**". Thus bacteria pathogenic for humans usually grow at 37°C (normal body temperature).

2. Oxygen

Based on their O_2 requirements, prokaryotes can be classified into aerobes and anaerobes.
A. **Aerobic bacteria**—require oxygen for growth and may be:
   i. *Obligate aerobes*—have an absolute or obligate requirement for oxygen, such as vibrio.
   i. *Facultative anaerobes*—are ordinarily aerobic but can also grow in the absence of oxygen, though less abundantly.
   iii. *Microaerophilic organisms*—grow best at low oxygen tension.
B. **Anaerobic bacteria**—grow in absence of oxygen.
   i. *Obligate anaerobes*—may even die on exposure to oxygen. For example, *Clostridium tetani*.

3. Carbon Dioxide

All bacteria require small amount of carbon dioxide for growth.

4. Moisture and Drying

Moisture is very essential for the growth of the bacteria.

5. pH

Most bacteria can live and multiply within the range of pH 5 (acidic) to pH 8 (basic) and have a pH optimum near neutral (pH 7).

6. Light

Darkness provides a favorable condition for growth and viability of bacteria.

7. Osmotic Effect
Bacteria are more tolerant to osmotic variation.

8. Mechanical and Sonic Stresses
In spite of tough walls of bacteria, they may be ruptured by mechanical stress.

KEY POINTS

- **Bacterial growth curve:** The bacterial growth curve can be divided into four major phases: lag phase, exponential or log (logarithmic) phase, stationary phase, and decline phase.
- The requirements for microbial growth—chemical and physical.

IMPORTANT QUESTIONS

1. Draw and describe a typical bacterial growth curve.
2. Write short notes on:
   a. Bacterial growth curve/Growth phases of bacteria.
   b. Physical factors influencing microbial growth.

MULTIPLE CHOICE QUESTIONS (MCQs)

1. Generation time for *Mycobacterium tuberculosis* is:
   a. 20 seconds   b. 20 minutes
   c. 20 hours   d. 20 days
2. Bacteria which can grow at temperature between 20 and 40°C are known as:
   a. Mesophiles   b. Psychrophiles
   c. Thermophiles d. None of the above
3. The bacteria which require much higher level of carbon dioxide for their growth are known as:
   a. Microaerophilic bacteria   b. Capnophilic bacteria
   c. Aerobic bacteria   d. Phototrophs
4. Which one of the following acidophilic bacteria can grow in acidic conditions?
   a. Escherichia coli   *b. Lactobacilli*
   c. Pseudomonas aeruginosa   *d. Vibrio cholerae*

Section 2: Microorganisms

5. The enzyme catalase is present in:
   a. Aerobic bacteria
   b. Obligate anaerobic bacteria
   c. Aerobic and obligate anaerobic bacteria
   d. None of the above

ANSWERS

1. c   2. a   3. b   4. b   5. a

CHAPTER 4

Normal Microbial Flora of the Human Body

Learning Objectives

After reading and studying this chapter, you should be able to:
❖ Describe role of normal flora in human body.
❖ List of organisms present as normal flora of upper respiratory tract, gastrointestinal tract and genitourinary tract.

■ INTRODUCTION

The term **"normal microbial flora"** denotes the population of microorganisms that inhabit the skin and mucous membranes of healthy normal persons.

■ NORMAL FLORA OF THE SKIN

The predominant resident microorganisms of the skin are aerobic and anaerobic diphtheroid bacilli (e.g., *Corynebacterium, Propionibacterium*); nonhemolytic aerobic and anaerobic staphylococci [*Staphylococcus epidermidis,* occasionally *Staphylococcus* (*S*) *aureus,* and *Peptostreptococcus* species]; gram-positive, aerobic, spore-forming bacilli that are ubiquitous in air, water, and soil; alpha hemolytic streptococci (viridans streptococci) and enterococci (*Enterococcus* species); and gram-negative coliform bacilli and *Acinetobacter*. Fungi and yeasts are often present in skin folds; acid-fast, nonpathogenic mycobacteria occur in areas rich in sebaceous secretions (genitalia, external ear). Hair frequently harbors *S. aureus* and forms a reservoir for cross infection.

■ NORMAL FLORA OF THE CONJUNCTIVA

The predominant organisms of the conjunctiva are diphtheroids (*Corynebacterium xerosis*), *S. epidermidis,* and nonhemolytic streptococci. *Neisseria* and gram-negative bacilli resembling hemophili (*Moraxella* species) are also frequently present. The conjunctival flora is normally held in cheek by the flow of tears, which contain antibacterial lysozyme.

■ NORMAL FLORA OF THE NOSE, NASOPHARYNX AND ACCESSORY SINUSES

The floor of the nose harbors *Corynebacteria, Staphylococci, Streptococci and Haemophilus* species and *Moraxella lacunata* may also be seen.

The nasopharynx of the infant is sterile at birth but, within 2-3 days after birth, acquires the common commensal flora and the pathogenic flora carried by the mother and the attendants. Certain gram-negative organisms from the intestinal tract such as *Pseudomonas aeruginosa, E. coli,* paracolons and *Proteus* are also occasionally found in normal persons. After penicillin therapy, they may be the predominant flora.

■ NORMAL FLORA OF THE MOUTH

The mucous membranes of the mouth and pharynx are often sterile at birth but may be contaminated by passage through the birth canal. Within 4-12 hours after birth, viridans streptococci become established as the most prominent members of the resident flora and remain so for life. They probably originate in the respiratory tracts of the mother and attendants. Early in life, aerobic and anaerobic staphylococci, gram-negative diplococci (*Neisseria, Moraxella catarrhalis),* diphtheroids, and occasional lactobacilli are added. When teeth begin to erupt, the anaerobic spirochetes, *Prevotella* species (especially *P. melaninogenica), Fusobacterium* species, *Rothia* species, and *Capnocytophaga* species establish themselves, along with some anaerobic vibrios and lactobacilli. Yeasts (*Candida* species) occur in the mouth.

■ NORMAL FLORA OF THE UPPER RESPIRATORY TRACT

Within 12 hours after birth, alpha hemolytic streptococci are found in the upper respiratory tract and become the dominant organisms of the oropharynx and remain so for life. Small bronchi and alveoli are normally sterile. In the pharynx and trachea, flora similar to that of the mouth establish themselves. The predominant organisms in the upper respiratory tract, particularly the pharynx, are nonhemolytic.

■ NORMAL FLORA OF THE GASTROINTESTINAL TRACT

At birth: At birth the intestine is sterile, but organisms are soon introduced with food. In all cases, within 4–24 hours of birth an intestinal flora is established partly from below and partly by invasion from above.

Breastfed children: In breastfed children the intestine contains lactobacilli *(L. bifidus)*, enterococci, colon bacilli and staphylococci. In artificially fed (bottle fed) children intestine contains *L. acidophilus* and colon bacilli and in part by enterococci, gram-positive aerobic and anaerobic bacilli.

Normal adult: Because of the low pH of the stomach, it is virtually sterile except soon after eating. The stomach's acidity keeps the number of microorganisms at a minimum.

As the pH of intestinal content becomes alkaline, the resident flora gradually increases. In the adult duodenum, there are 10^3–10^6 bacteria per gram of content; in the jejunum and ileum, 10^5–10^8 bacteria per gram; and in the cecum and transverse colon, 10^8–10^{10} bacteria per gram. In the upper intestine, lactobacilli and enterococci predominate, but in the lower ileum and cecum, the flora is fecal. In the sigmoid colon and rectum, there are about 10^{11} bacteria per gram of contents, constituting 10–30% of the fecal mass.

In the normal adult colon, 96–99% of the resident bacterial flora consists of anaerobes: *Bacteroides* species, especially *B. fragilis*; *Fusobacterium* species; anaerobic lactobacilli, e.g., bifidobacteria; clostridia (*C. perfringens*, 10^3–10^5/g); and anaerobic gram-positive cocci (*Peptostreptococcus* species). Only 1–4% are facultative aerobes.

■ NORMAL FLORA OF THE GENITOURINARY TRACT

Mycobacterium smegmatis, a harmless commensal, is found in the smegma of the genitalia of both men and women. From apparently normal men, aerobic and anaerobic bacteria can be cultured from a high proportion, including lactobacilli, *Gardnerella vaginalis*, alpha hemolytic streptococci and *Bacteroides species*. *Chlamydia trachomatis* and *Ureaplasma urealyticum* may also be present. The female urethra is either sterile or contains a few gram-positive cocci.

Female vaginal area: The female vaginal area has an acid pH between puberty and menopause, but the secretions are alkaline at other times.

At birth: At birth the vagina is sterile. In the first 24 hours it is invaded by micrococci, enterococci and diphtheroids. In 2–3 days, the maternal estrin induces glycogen deposition in the vaginal epithelium. This facilitates the growth of a lactobacillus (Doderlien's bacillus) which produces acid from glycogen, and the flora for a few weeks is similar to that of the adult. After the passively transferred estrin has been eliminated in the urine, the glycogen disappears, along with Doderlien's bacillus and the pH of the vagina becomes alkaline. This brings about a change in the flora to micrococci, alpha and nonhemolytic streptococci, coliforms and diphtheroids.

At puberty: At puberty, the glycogen reappears and the pH changes to acid due to the metabolic activity of Doderlien's bacilli, *E. coli* and yeasts. This appears to be an important mechanism in preventing the establishment of other, possibly harmful microorganisms in the vagina. During pregnancy there is an increase in *Staphylococcus epidermidis,* Doderlien's bacilli, and yeasts. After menopause, lactobacilli again diminish in number and a mixed flora returns and the flora resembles that found before puberty.

KEY POINT

The term "normal microbial flora" denotes the population of microorganisms that inhabit the skin and mucous membrane of normal healthy individuals.

IMPORTANT QUESTIONS

1. What is normal microbial flora of the human body? Write briefly on role of normal flora in human body.
2. Write short notes on:
   a. Normal bacterial flora.
   b. Normal flora in the mouth and upper respiratory tract.
   c. Normal flora of the genitourinary tract.

MULTIPLE CHOICE QUESTIONS (MCQs)

1. The majority of normal bacteria flora are present in:
   a. Conjunctiva
   b. Skin
   c. Nasopharynx
   d. Large intestine
2. Which bacteria is responsible for producing acidic pH in adult vagina?
   a. *Lactobacillus*
   b. *Bacteroides* species
   c. Diphtheroids
   d. *Gardnerella vaginalis*

ANSWERS

1. d   2. a

CHAPTER 5

Pathogenesis and Common Diseases

Learning Objectives

After reading and studying this chapter, you should be able to:
- List human diseases caused by bacteria, viruses, fungi and parasites.

■ COMMON DISEASES CAUSED BY DIFFERENT MICROORGANISMS

Infectious Agent

Pathogenic microorganisms are infectious agents. These pathogens vary among bacteria, viruses, fungi, and parasites. All these microorganisms require food for growth and a suitable environment to live. The strength of the microorganism, the number of microorganisms present, the effectiveness of a person's immune system, and the length of exposure to the microorganisms determine a pathogen's ability to produce disease.

■ HUMAN DISEASES CAUSED BY BACTERIA

Knowing the type of organism is important to the treatment of the patient. With many diseases, proper diagnosis and treatment are not possible until the specific microorganism causing the illness has been identified **(Table 5.1)**.

TABLE 5.1: Human diseases caused by bacteria.		
Type	**Species**	**Disease**
Gram-positive cocci	*Staphylococcus aureus*	**Cutaneous infections:** Folliculitis, boils, carbuncles, impetigo, and purulent abscesses. These cutaneous infections can progress to **deeper abscesses** involving

Contd...

Contd...

Type	Species	Disease
		other organ systems and progress to septicemia and bacteremia. **Toxin-induced diseases:** Food poisoning, scalded skin syndrome (SSS), toxic shock syndrome (TSS) **Other systemic diseases:** Bacteremia include pneumonia, empyema, septic arthritis, osteomyelitis, acute endocarditis, and catheter-related bacteremia

	Streptococcus pyogenes	**A. Respiratory infection**
		  i. Streptococcal pharyngitis
		  ii. Scarlet fever
		B. Pyogenic cutaneous infections: impetigo, erysipelas, cellulitis, necrotizing fasciitis involving deep subcutaneous tissues, streptococcal toxic shock syndrome
		Nonsuppurative sequelae: Rheumatic fever and acute glomerulonephritis.

	Streptococcus pneumoniae	Pneumonia, meningitis, sinusitis and otitis media, bacteremia, and endocarditis
Gram-negative cocci	Neisseria meningitis	Meningitis, meningoencephalitis, bacteremia, pneumonia, arthritis, urethritis
	Neisseria gonorrhoeae	Urethritis, cervicitis, salpingitis, pelvic inflammatory disease, proctitis, bacteremia, arthritis, conjunctivitis, and pharyngitis
Gram-positive bacilli	C. diphtheriae	❖ Diphtheria occurs in two forms **(respiratory and cutaneous)** ❖ A tough gray to white pseudomembrane, may appear on the tonsils and then spread downward into the larynx and trachea ❖ **Systemic effects** involving the **kidneys, heart, and nervous** system ❖ **In cutaneous diphtheria,** systemic complications are less common **Complications:** 1. Asphyxia 2. Acute circulatory failure 3. Postdiphtheritic paralysis 4. **Septic, such as pneumonia and otitis media**
	Bacillus anthracis	Emetic (vomiting) and diarrheal forms of gastroenteritis; ocular infection, other opportunistic infections
	Clostridium perfringens	1. Soft tissue infections (cellulitis, suppurative myositis, myonecrosis) 2. Food poisoning 3. Septicemia

Contd...

Contd...

Type	Species	Disease
	Clostridium tetani	Tetanus
	Clostridium botulinum	**Botulism:** It is of three types—foodborne botulism, wound botulism, and infant botulism
	Clostridium difficile	1. A symptomatic colonization 2. Antibiotic-associated diarrhea (AAD) 3. Pseudomembranous colitis
Gram-negative rods	*Escherichia coli*	1. **Urinary tract infection**; limited to bladder (cystitis) or can spread to kidneys (pyelonephritis) or prostate (prostatitis) 2. **Diarrhea:** EHEC is an important cause of hemorrhagic colitis (HC) and hemolytic uremic syndrome (HUS) in the United States 3. **Pyogenic infections:** Neonatal meningitis 4. **Bacteremia**
	Klebsiella pneumoniae	Primary community-acquired pnuemonia, nosocomial infections, urinary tract infections, wound infections, bacteremia and meningitis and rarely diarrhea
	Proteus spp.	Urinary tract infections, wound infections, pneumonia
	Shigella dysenteriae	❖ Bacillary dysentery (Shigellosis) ❖ Hemolytic colitis and hemolytic uremic syndrome (HUS)
	Salmonella spp.	❖ Asymptomatic colonization (primarily with *S. typhi* and *S. paratyphi*) ❖ Enteric fever also called typhoid fever (*S. typhi*) or paratyphoid fever (*S. paratyphi*) ❖ Enteritis—characterized by fever, nausea, vomiting, bloody or nonbloody diarrhea, and abdominal cramps ❖ Bacteremia
	Vibrio cholerae	❖ Cholera
	Campylobacter spp.	**Zoonotic infection**; gastroenteritis, septicemia, meningitis, spontaneous abortion, proctitis, Guillain–Barre syndrome, septicemia and is disseminated to multiple organs
	Helicobacter pylori	Gastritis, peptic ulcers, gastric adenocarcinoma
	Pseudomonas aeruginosa	A. **Community infections:** 1. Otitis externa and varicose ulcers 2. Corneal infections

Contd...

Contd...

Type	Species	Disease

		3. Jacuzzi rash or whirlpool rash
		4. Industrial eye injuries
		B. **Hospital infections:**
		  1. Localized lesions
		  2. Septicemia and endocarditis
		  3. Ecthyma gangrenosum and many other types of skin lesions
		  4. Infection of the nail bed
		  5. Infantile diarrhea and sepsis
		  6. Shanghai fever
		  7. Other infections: Gastrointestinal tract, central nervous system, and musculoskeletal system
		P. aeruginosa is regularly a cause of nosocomial pneumonia, nosocomial urinary tract infections, surgical site infections, infections of severe burns and infections of patients undergoing either chemotherapy for neoplastic diseases or **antibiotic therapy**

	Burkholderia cepacia	Respiratory tract infections, particularly in patients with cystic fibrosis; urinary tract infections; septic arthritis; peritonitis; septicemia; opportunistic infections
	Burkholderia pseudomallei	Asymptomatic colonization; cutaneous infection with regional lymphadenitis, fever, and malaise; pulmonary disease ranging from bronchitis to necrotizing pneumonia
	Burkholderia mallei	Glanders in livestock
	Legionella pneumophila	Legionnaires disease, a life-threatening multifocal pneumonia; pontiac fever, a self-limited, febrile, flu-like illness
	Yersinia pestis *Pasteurella multocida*	Plague 1. Local abscess at the site of a cat or dog bite 2. Infarctions of the respiratory system 3. Meningitis or cerebral abscess
	Francisella tularensis	Tularemia (rabbit fever)
	Haemophilus influenzae *Haemophilus ducreyi*	Meningitis, epiglottitis, cellulitis, arthritis, otitis, sinusitis, lower respiratory tract disease, conjunctivitis
	Haemophilus influenzae biogroup aegyptius *Haemophilus ducreyi*	Purulent conjunctivitis and Brazilian purpuric fever (BPF). Sexually transmitted disease (STD) chancroid or soft sore

Contd...

Contd...

Type	Species	Disease
	Bordetella pertussis	Whooping cough
	Brucella melitensis	Brucellosis
	Mycobacterium tuberculosis	**Pulmonary tuberculosis** Complications include miliary tuberculosis, disseminated tuberculosis, tubercular meningitis, tuberculosis of the skin, tuberculosis of the middle ear and ocular structures
	Atypical mycobacteria	(A) Localized lymphadenitis; (B) Skin lesions following traumatic inoculation of bacteria; (C) Tuberculosis-like pulmonary lesions; (D) Disseminated disease
	Mycobacterium leprae	Leprosy
	Spirochetes Treponema pallidum Borrelia recurrentis Borrelia burgdorferi Leptospira interrogans-	Syphilis Relapsing fever Lyme disease Leptospirosis
	Mycoplasma Ureaplasma	*Mycoplasma pneumonia:* Primary atypical pneumonia
	Actinomycetes	Actinomycosis
	Miscellaneous bacteria	
	Listeria monocytogenes	Septicemia and meningitis are the most common forms of listeriosis. Intrauterine infection of the fetus may result in abortion, stillbirth, remature delivery, or acute-onset disseminated infection in the newborn infant (including the form known as granulomatosis infantisepticum). Asymptomatic infection of the female genital tract may cause infertility. Meningitis or septicemia may occur in neonates.
	Erysipelothrix rhusiopathiae	Three forms of human infection—(1) **erysipeloid,** (2) **generalized cutaneous form and** (3) **septicemia**
	Alcaligenes faecalis	Urinary tract infection, infantile gastroenteritis, and typhoid-like fever in humans
	Chromobacterium violaceum	Intestinal and genitourinary infections and septicemic illnesses with pneumonia
	Flavobacterium meningosepticum	Opportunistic infections, neonatal meningitis in premature infants and pneumonia in immunocompromised hosts

Contd...

Contd...

Type	Species	Disease
	Calymmatobacterium (donovania) granulomatis	Granuloma inguinale, a sexually transmitted disease
	Acinetobacter species	Nosocomial infections
	Streptobacillus moniliformis and Spirillum minus	Rat bite fever
	Eikenella corrodens	In the settings of a human bite wound or fistfight injury. Other infections are endocarditis, sinusitis, meningitis, brain abscesses, pneumonia, and lung abscesses
	Cardiobacterium hominis	Endocarditis
	Capnocytophaga species	Severe periodontal disease in juveniles, bacteremia and severe systemic disease in immunocompromised patients
	Gardnerella vaginalis	Bacterial vaginosis
	Rickettsiaceae and Bartonellaceae	Rickettsia rickettsiae—rocky mountain spotted fever
	Chlamydia and Chlamydophila Chlamydia trachomatis Chlamydia psittaci Chlamydophila pneumoniae	Trachoma Ornithosis (Psittacosis) Pneumonia

■ HUMAN DISEASES CAUSED BY FUNGI

Fungal (mycotic) infections are among the most common diseases found in humans.

Mycotic infections are diseases caused by yeasts and molds. Some are superficial, involving the skin and the mucous membranes. Most frequently, the infections involve the external layers of the skin, the hair, and the nails and are commonly referred to as ringworm (dermatomycosis). Other common sites include men's beards (barber's itch), the feet (athlete's foot), and around the nails. Domestic pets sometimes have ringworm infection and are frequently the source of infection for humans **(Table 5.2)**.

Fungi also invade the deeper tissues of the body at times. Most of these infections produce no signs or symptoms; however, some become serious and potentially fatal, especially in a patient who is severely immunocompromised, such as coccidioidomycosis (valley fever) and histoplasmosis (a systemic fungal respiratory disease).

Mycoses (Fungus Infections)

Infection caused by fungus is known as mycosis (plural: mycoses). Classification of fungal disease according to primary sites of infections is given in **Table 5.2**.

TABLE 5.2: Classification of fungal disease according to primary sites of infections.

Type of mycosis	Causative fungal agents	Mycosis
A. Superficial	Malassezia species	Pityriasis versicolor
	Hortaea werneckii	Tinea nigra
	Trichosporon species	White piedra
	Piedraia hortae	Black piedra
B. Cutaneous	Microsporum species, trichophyton species, and Epidermophyton floccosum	Dermatophytosis
	Candida albicans and other candida species	Candidiasis of skin, mucosa, or nails
C. Subcutaneous	Sporothrix schenckii Phialophora verrucosa, Fonsecaea pedrosoi, others	Sporotrichosis Chromoblastomycosis
	Pseudallescheria boydii, Madurella mycetomatis, others	Mycetoma
	Exophiala, bipolaris, exserohilum, and others	Phaeohyphomycosis
D. Systemic (primary, endemic)	Coccidioides immitis, C. posadasii Histoplasma capsulatum Blastomyces dermatitidis Paracoccidioides brasiliensis	Coccidioidomycosis Histoplasmosis Blastomycosis Paracoccidioidomycosis
E. Opportunistic	Candida albicans and other candida species	Systemic candidiasis
	Cryptococcus neoformans	Cryptococcosis
	Aspergillus fumigatus and other aspergillus species	Aspergillosis
	Species of Rhizopus, Absidia, Mucor, and other zygomycetes	Mucormycosis (zygomycosis)
	Penicillium marneffei	Penicilliosis

■ HUMAN DISEASES CAUSED BY PARASITES (TABLES 5.3 AND 5.4)

TABLE 5.3: Human diseases caused by parasites.

Phylum	Pathogen	Disease
Amoebozoa (amebae)	Entamoeba histolytica	Amoebic dysentery
	Acanthamoeba species	Amoebic keratitis
Metamonada (flagellates)	Giardia lamblia (Giardia intestinalis)	Giardiasis
Parabasala (flagellates)	Trichomonas vaginalis	Protozoal vaginitis
Eulenozoa (flagellates)	Trypanosoma brucei	African sleeping sickness
	Trypanosoma cruzi	Chaga's disease
	Leishmania donovani	Kala azar
Apicomplexa (sporozoans)	Plasmodium spp.(Plasmodium falciparum, Plasmodium malariae, Plasmodium ovale, and Plasmodium vivax)	Malaria
	Babesia spp.	Babesial infection (babesiosis)
	Toxoplasma gondii	Toxoplasmosis
	Crytptosporidium spp.	Cryptosporidiosis
Ciliophora (ciliates)	Balantidium coli	Balantidial dysentery

TABLE 5.4: Human diseases caused by helminthes.

Phylum	Pathogen	Disease
Platyhelminthes	Paragonimus westermanni (lung fluke)	Paragonimiasis
	Schistosoma sp. (blood flukes)	Schistosomiasis
	Clonorchis sinensis (Chinese liver fluke)	Clonorchiasis
	Taenia saginata (beef tapeworm)	Taeniasis
	Taenia solium (pork tapeworm)	Taeniasis
	Hymenolepis nana (dwarf tapeworm)	Hymenolepiasis
	Diphyllobothrium latum (fish tapeworm)	Diphyllobothriasis
	Echinococcus granulosus (dog tapeworm)	Echinococcosis
	Fasciola hepatica (sheep liver fluke)	Fascioliasis

Contd...

Contd...

Phylum	Pathogen	Disease
Nematoda (roundworms)	*Strongyloides stercoralis* (threadworm)	Strongyloidiasis
	Ascaris lumbricoides (roundworm)	Ascariasis
	Necator americanus (hookworm)	New world hookworm disease
	Ancylostoma duodenale	Old world hookworm disease (hookworm)
	Enterobius vermicularis (pinworm)	Pinworm feotalism
	Trichuris trichiura (whipworm)	Trichuriasis
	Trichinella spiralis (trichina worm)	Trichinosis
	Wuchereria bancrofti	Elephantiasis or bancroftian filariasis
	Dirofilaria immitis (heartworm)	Filariasis

■ VIRUSES

The human diseases caused by DNA viruses are listed in **Table 5.5** and the RNA viruses are listed in **Table 5.6**.

TABLE 5.5: Human diseases caused by DNA viruses.

Family	Viruses	Disease
1. Poxviridae family	Smallpox virus	Smallpox
2. Herpesviridae	Herpes viruses	HSV-1 causes acute herpetic gingivostomatitis, acute herpetic pharyngotonsillitis, herpes labialis, herpes encephalitis, eczema herpeticum, and herpetic whitlow. HSV-2 causes genital herpes, neonatal infection, and aseptic meningitis. **Varicella zoster virus (VZV)** causes chickenpox (varicella) and herpes zoster or shingles, two distinct clinical entities in humans.
	Cytomegalovirus	Mononucleosis syndrome in immunocompetent hosts. Congenital CMV infection, acquired CMV infection, CMV infection in immunocompromised patients, and CMV infection in immunocompetent adult hosts. CMV generally causes subclinical infection

Contd...

Contd...

Family	Viruses	Disease
	Epstein-Barr virus	Infectious mononucleosis, Burkitt's lymphoma, Hodgkin's disease, and nasopharyngeal carcinoma.
3. Adenoviridae		A. Respiratory diseases 　1. Pharyngitis 　2. Pneumonia 　3. Acute respiratory diseases (ARD) B. Eye infections 　1. Pharyngoconjunctival fever 　2. Epidemic keratoconjunctivitis (EKC) 　3. Acute follicular conjunctivitis C. Diarrhea D. Mesenteric adenitis and intussusception in children
4. Papovaviridae family	**Papovaviruses:** *Papillomavirus* *Polyomavirus*	Papillomaviruses cause several different kinds of warts in humans, including cutaneous warts, genital warts, respiratory papillomatosis, oral papillomas, and cancer. Till date, no documented association with any naturally occurring tumor of man
5. Parvoviridae	1. **Parvoviruses** 2. **Dependovirus** 3. **Erythrovirus**	None pathogenic in humans None pathogenic in humans Respiratory infection with an erythematous maculopapular rash [erythema infectiosum (slapped cheek disease), joint disease, aplastic crisis in children with chronic hemolytic anemia (sickle cell disease), nonimmune fetal hydrops following infection during pregnancy and persistent anemia in immunodeficients]'
6. Hepadnaviridae family	Hepatitis type B virus	Hepatitis B (serum hepatitis)

TABLE 5.6: Human diseases caused by RNA viruses.

Family	Viruses	Disease
Picornaviridae	Poliovirus	Polio
	Coxsackievirus	Herpangina (vesicular pharyngitis), aseptic meningitis, hand-foot-and-mouth disease, respiratory infections, epidemic myalgia or Bornholm

Contd...

Contd...

Family	Viruses	Disease
		disease, myocardial and pericardial infections, Juvenile diabetes, neonatal infections, chronic fatigue syndrome
	Echoviruses	1. Aseptic meningitis 2. Respiratory illnesses in children 3. Infantile diarrhea 4. Occasionally, conjunctivitis, muscle weakness, and spasm
	Hepatitis A virus	Hepatitis (infectious hepatitis)
	Rhinovirus	❖ Common cold ❖ Upper respiratory tract infections
Orthomyxoviridae	Influenza virus types A, B, and C	Influenza
Paramyxoviridae	Parainfluenza virus	Respiratory tract syndromes ranging from a **mild cold-like upper respiratory tract infection** (coryza, pharyngitis, mild bronchitis, wheezing, and fever) to **bronchiolitis and** pneumonia
	Measles virus	Measles, atypical measles, and subacute sclerosing panencephalitis (SSPE)
	Mumps virus	Mumps
	Respiratory syncytial virus	Common cold to pneumonia
Togaviridae	Rubella virus	Rubella
	Western, eastern, and Venezuelan equine encephalitis virus	Encephalitis in horses and humans
	Ross River virus	Epidemic polyarthritis
	Sindbis virus	No association with human diseases
	Semliki Forest virus	No association with human disease
Flaviviridae	Yellow fever virus	Yellow fever
	Dengue virus	Dengue fever
	St. Louis encephalitis virus	Mild febrile illness to frank encephalitis
	Hepatitis C virus	Acute hepatitis; chronic persistent infection; severe rapid progression to cirrhosis

Contd...

Contd...

Family	Viruses	Disease
Bunyaviridae	California encephalitis virus	Encephalitis, aseptic meningitis and fever
	LaCrosse virus	Encephalitis, aseptic meningitis and fever
	Sandfly fever virus	Pappataci fever (three day fever)
	Crimean Congo hemorrhagic fever virus	Fever, myalgia, (muscle ache), dizziness, neck pain and stiffness, backache, headache, sore eyes and photophobia (sensitivity to light). There may be nausea, vomiting, diarrhea, abdominal pain and sore throat early on, followed by sharp mood swings and confusion
	Hanta virus	Hemorrhagic fever with renal syndrome
Arenaviridae	Lymphocytic choriomeningitis virus	Lymphocytic choriomeningitis
	Lassa fever virus	Lassa fever
	Tacaribe group of Arenavirus complex (Junin, Guanarito Machupo, and Sabia viruses)	South American hemorrhagic fever
Rhabdoviridae	Rabies virus	Rabies
Reoviridae	Rotavirus	Diarrhea in infants and children
	Colorado tick fever virus	Mountain fever or tick fever
Coronaviridae	Coronavirus	Common colds, gastroenteritis in infants; severe acute respiratory syndrome (SARS)
Retroviridae	Human T-cell leukemia virus types I	Adult T-cell leukemia/lymphoma
	Human immunodeficiency virus-1 and 2	Acquired immunodeficiency syndrome (AIDS)
Caliciviridae	Norwalk virus	Epidemic viral gastroenteritis in adults
	Hepevirus-Hepatitis E virus	Acute hepatitis including jaundice, chronic hepatitis cirrhosis, hepatocellular carcinoma

Contd...

Contd...

Family	Viruses	Disease
Filoviridae	Ebola virus	Hemorrhagic fever
	Marburg virus	Hemorrhagic fever

The families of RNA viruses and some important members are described in **Table 5.7**.

TABLE 5.7: Families of RNA viruses and some important members.

Family	Members
Picornaviridae	Rhinoviruses, *poliovirus*, echoviruses, coxsackievirus, hepatitis A virus
Orthomyxoviridae	*Influenza virus* types A, B, and C
Paramyxoviridae	Parainfluenza virus, Sendai virus, *measles virus*, mumps virus, respiratory syncytial virus
Togaviridae	*Rubella virus;* western, eastern, and Venezuelan equine encephalitis virus; Ross River virus; Sindbis virus; Semliki forest virus
Flaviviridae	*Yellow fever virus,* dengue virus, St. Louis encephalitis virus, hepatitis C virus
Bunyaviridae	*California encephalitis virus,* La Crosse virus, sandfly fever virus, hemorrhagic fever virus, Hanta virus
Arenaviridae	*Lassa fever virus,* Tacaribe virus complex, Junin and Machupo viruses, lymphocytic choriomeningitis virus
Rhabdoviridae	*Rabies virus,* vesicular stomatitis virus, *Ebola virus,* Marburg virus
Reoviridae	*Rotavirus,* Colorado tick fever virus
Coronaviridae	Coronavirus
Retroviridae	Human T-cell leukemia virus types I and II, *human immunodeficiency virus,* animal oncoviruses
Caliciviridae	Norwalk virus, Delta agent
Filoviridae	*Ebola virus,* Marburg virus

KEY POINTS

Pathogenic microorganisms are infectious agents. These pathogens vary among bacteria, viruses, yeasts, fungi, and protozoa. Human infections caused by gram-positive and gram-negative cocci and gram-positive and gram-negative bacilli. Mycotic infections are diseases caused by yeasts and molds. Human diseases caused by parasites such as protozoa, helminths and by virus (DNA viruses and RNA viruses).

Chapter 5: Pathogenesis and Common Diseases

IMPORTANT QUESTIONS
1. Name various diseases caused by gram-positive cocci.
2. Name various diseases caused by gram-negative cocci.
3. Name various diseases caused by gram-positive bacilli.
4. Name various diseases caused by gram-negative bacilli.
5. Name various diseases caused by protozoa and helminthes.
6. Name various diseases caused by DNA viruses.
7. Name various diseases caused by RNA viruses.

MULTIPLE CHOICE QUESTIONS (MCQs)
1. Which of the following bacteria can cause gonorrhea?
   a. *Neisseria gonorrhoeae*
   b. *Stretococcus pyogenes*
   c. *Staphylococcus aureus*
   d. *Clostridium tetani*
2. Pulmonary tuberculosis is caused by the following bacteria:
   a. *Staphylococcus aureus*
   b. *Mycobacteria tuberculosis*
   c. *Staphylococcus aureus*
   d. *Escherichia coli*
3. Which of the following fungi is causative agent of cryptococcosis?
   a. *Aspergillus fumigatus*
   b. *Cryptococcus neoformans*
   c. *Candida albicans*
   d. None of the above
4. *Histoplasma capsulatum* is the causative agent of:
   a. Histoplasmosis
   b. Cryptococcosis
   c. Aspergillosis
   d. None of the above
5. *Entamoeba histolytica* is the causative agent of:
   a. Amoebic dysentery
   b. Dengue fever
   c. Enteric fever
   d. None of the above
6. Which of the following parasite can cause Ascariasis?
   a. *Trichinella spiralis*
   b. *Nector americans*
   c. *Ascaris lumbricoides*
   d. None of the above
7. Rabies virus is the causative agent of:
   a. Yellow fever
   b. Dengue fever
   c. Influenza
   d. Rabies
8. Which of the following viruses can cause hepatitis?
   a. Hepatitis A virus
   b. Hepatitis B virus
   c. All of the above
   d. None of the above

ANSWERS
| 1. a | 2. b | 3. b | 4. a | 5. a | 6. c |
| 7. d | 8. c | | | | |

CHAPTER 6

Methods for Study of Microbes

Learning Objectives

After reading and studying this chapter, you should be able to:
- Describe universal precautions.
- Discuss identification of microorganisms from specimens.

■ INTRODUCTION

The major focus of the clinical microbiologist is to isolate and identify microorganisms from clinical specimen accurately and rapidly.

■ METHODS FOR STUDY OF MICROBES

Identification of microorganisms from specimens is based on: (1) microscopic examination of specimens; (2) growth and biochemical characteristics of microorganisms isolated from cultures; and (3) immunologic technique that detect antibodies or microbial antigens.

1. Microscopy

Wet-mount, heat-fixed, or chemically fixed specimens can be examined with an ordinary bright-field microscope. For bacteriology, the Gram and Ziehl-Neelsen stains are usually sufficient, but for the demonstration of fungi or parasites special stains or concentration techniques may be required.

"**Wet**" **mounts**, i.e., unstained preparations of fluid material, are widely used in looking at cells in urine, cerebrospinal fluid (CSF), feces, and vaginal secretions. They are ideal rapid methods (takes >5 or 10 min). Similarly, a rapid diagnosis of falciparum malaria can be life-saving. Indeed, suspected **pyogenic meningitis** and **falciparum malaria** are among the few conditions for which it is clearly justifiable to call upon emergency laboratory services outside normal working hours.

Electron microscopy is much slower and is valuable in the relatively rapid diagnosis of certain viral infections, including viral diarrhea.

2. Culture Isolation and Identification of the Agent

Typically microorganisms have been identified by their particular growth patterns and biochemical characteristics. These characteristics vary depending on whether the clinical microbiologist is dealing with viruses, fungi (yeast, molds). Parasites (protozoa, helminths), common gram-positive or gram-negative bacteria, rickettsias, chlamydiae or mycoplasmas.

Principles

The principles remain the same: use sterile equipment and media (with cell lines if necessary) and add clinical material. After incubation at 37°C, for a variable time, from a few hours for enterobacteria to weeks for mycobacteria and some viruses and fungi, a visible effect will be produced. This might be colonies growing on agar or a cytopathic effect (CPE) in tissue culture. The skill of microbiology is in identifying the microbes responsible for the effect.

Identification

a. **Bacteria:** The presence of bacterial growth usually can be recognized by the development of colonies on solid media or turbidity in liquid media. Most pathogenic bacteria require only a few hours to produce visible growth whereas it may take weeks for colonies of **mycobacteria or mycoplasmas** to become evident.
   i. **Rickettsias:** Rickettsias can be diagnosed by immunoassays or by isolation of the microorganism. Immunological methods are preferred. Isolation of rickettsias and diagnosis of rickettsial diseases is generally confined to reference and specialized research laboratories.
   ii. **Chlamydiae:** Chlamydiae can be demonstrated in tissues and cell scrapings with Giemsa staining, which detects the characteristic intracellular inclusion bodies. Immunofluorescent staining of tissues and cells with

monoclonal antibody reagents is a more sensitive and specific means of diagnosis. The most sensitive methods for demonstrating Chlamydiae in clinical specimens are DNA probes and polymerase chain reaction (PCR) methods.
   iii. **Mycoplasmas:** The most routinely used techniques for identification of the mycoplasmas are immunological (hemagglutinin) or complement fixing antigen-antibody reactions using the patient's serum. These microorganisms are slow growing; therefore positive results from isolation procedure are rarely available before 30 days-a long delay with an approach that offers little advantage over standard techniques. Recently **DNA probes** have been applied to the detection of *Mycoplasma pneumoniae* in clinical specimens.

b. **Viruses:** Viruses are identified by isolation in conventional cell (tissue) culture by immunodiagnosis (fluorescent antibody, enzyme immunoassay, radioimmunoassay, latex agglutination. and immunoperoxidase) tests, and by molecular detection methods such as nucleic acid probes and amplification assays. Several types of systems are available for virus cultivation: cell cultures. embryonated hen's eggs, and experimental animals.

c. **Fungi:** Fungal infections often are diagnosed by:
   i. **Direct microscopic (fluorescence) examination of specimens.**
   ii. **Fungal cultures** remain as the standard for the recovery of fungi from patient specimens. However, the time needed to culture fungi varies anywhere from a few days to several weeks depending on the organism.
   iii. **Fungal serology: Fungal serology** (e.g., complement fixation and immunodiffusion) is designed to detect serum antibody but is limited to a few fungi *(Blastomyces dermatitidis, Coccidioides immitis, Histoplasma capsulatum)*. The cryptococcal latex antigen test is routinely used for the direct detection of *Cryptococcus neoformans* in serum and cerebrospinal fluid.
   iv. **Nonautomated (conventional kits) and automated methods:** In the clinical laboratory, nonautomated (conventional kits) and automated methods for rapid identification (4–24 hours) are used to detect most yeasts. Any biochemical methods used to detect fungi should always be accompanied by morphological studies examining for pseudohyphae, yeast cell structure, chlamydospores, and so on.

d. **Parasites:**
   i. **Concentrated wet mounts:** Concentrated wet mounts of blood, stool, or urine specimens can be examined microscopically for the presence of eggs, cysts, larvae, or vegetative cells of parasites.
   ii. **Blood smears:** Blood smears for **sporozoan (malaria)** and **flagellate (trypanosome) parasites** are stained with Giemsa. Some serological tests also are available.

3. Nonculture Methods

Antibodies labeled with fluorescent molecules are widely used in diagnostic virology, e.g., for respiratory secretions to find respiratory syncytial virus. Enzyme-linked immunosorbent assay (ELISA) kits are used for chlamydia detection, and many other *immunoprobes* are commercially produced or under investigation. DNA and RNA probes can be carried out with minimal expertise. Use of the **polymerase chain reaction** has greatly increased the sensitivity of nucleic acid probes.

4. Serology

Immunologic systems for the detection and identification of pathogens from clinical specimens are easy to use, give relatively rapid reaction endpoints, and are sensitive and specific (they give a low percentage of false positives and negatives). Serology is still the most common method of diagnosing the causes of "atypical" pneumonia (mycoplasmal pneumonia, psittacosis, Legionnaires' disease), syphilis, brucellosis and many viral infections, including human immunodeficiency virus (HIV). It is preferable to take a blood sample early in the illness (the *acute serum)* and another 10–14 days after the onset (the *convalescent serum);* a four-fold or greater rise in antibody titer in the second specimen is diagnostic of acute infection. With some infections, such as HIV and hepatitis B and C, much longer times must elapse.

5. Molecular Methods and Analysis of Metabolic Products

Some of the most accurate approaches to microbial identification are through the analysis of proteins and nucleic acids. Three methods being widely used are **nucleic acid probes, gas-liquid chromatography, and plasmid fingerprinting.**

6. Antimicrobial Sensitivity Testing

Determining the susceptibility of a microorganism to specific antibiotics is one of the most important tests performed in the clinical microbiology laboratory. Results can show the antibiotics to which a microorganism is most susceptible and the proper therapeutic dose needed to treat the infectious disease. Dilution susceptibility tests, disk diffusion tests (Kirby-Bauer method), the Etest strip and drug concentration measurements in the blood are used for testing.

KEY POINTS

- ❖ **Identification of microorganisms from specimens:** It is based on: (1) microscopic examination of specimens; (2) growth and biochemical characteristics of microorganisms isolated from cultures; and (3) immunologic technique that detect antibodies or microbial antigens.
- ❖ Viruses are identified by isolation in living cells (cell culture, embryonated hen's eggs, and experimental animals) or immunologic tests.
- ❖ Identification of fungi often can be made if a portion of the specimen is mixed with a drop of 10% Calcofluor White stain.
- ❖ Wet mounts of stool specimens or urine can be examined microscopically for the presence of parasites.
- ❖ Various molecular methods and analyses of metabolic products also can be used to identify microorganisms which include nucleic acid-based detection, gas-liquid chromatography, and plasmid fingerprinting.
- ❖ Susceptibility tests are used to find which method of control will be most effective.

IMPORTANT QUESTIONS

1. Write short notes on:
    a. Universal precautions
    b. Identification of microorganisms from specimens

Chapter 6: Methods for Study of Microbes

MULTIPLE CHOICE QUESTIONS (MCQs)

1. Bacteria that are most commonly transmitted by direct hand contact, causing nosocomial infection are:
   a. *Escherichia coli*
   b. *Enterococcus* species
   c. *Staphylococcus aureus*
   d. *Clostridium perfringens*
2. Hospital-associated respiratory infections are caused by which of the following bacteria?
   a. *Staphylococcus aureus*
   b. *Klebsiella*
   c. *Enterobacter*
   d. All of the above

ANSWERS
1. c   2. d

CHAPTER 7

Culture Media and Culture Methods

Learning Objectives

After reading and studying this chapter, you should be able to:
- Describe classification of media.
- Differentiate between the following: Enriched media and enrichment media; indicator media and differential media; selective media and differential media with suitable examples.
- Discuss liquid media with its composition and uses.
- Discuss anaerobic culture methods.
- Explain the principle and describe uses of the following: McIntosh and Fildes anaerobic jar; cooked meat broth.

■ INTRODUCTION

Culture medium: A nutrient material prepared for the growth of microorganisms in a laboratory is called a **culture medium.**

■ CLASSIFICATION OF MEDIA

Media have been classified in many ways **(Box 7.1)**.

A. Phases of Growth Media

Growth media are used in either of two phases: Liquid (broth) or solid (agar).

B. Based on Nutritional Factors

1. *Simple Media (Basal Media)*

Simple media are those which contain only basic nutrients, *e.g.*, peptone water, nutrient broth, and nutrient agar. These simple media

> **Box 7.1:** Classification of media.
>
> **A. Based on phases of growth media**
>   1. Liquid (broth) media
>   2. Solid (agar) media
>   3. Semisolid media
>
> **B. Based on nutritional factors**
>   1. Simple media (basal media)
>   2. Complex media
>   3. Synthetic or defined media
>
> **C. Special media**
>   1. Enriched media
>   2. Enrichment media
>   3. Selective media
>   4. Indicator or differential media
>   5. Transport media
>   6. Sugar media
>
> **D. Reducing media**
>   Based on phases of growth media
>   1. Liquid (broth) media
>   2. Solid (agar) media
>   3. Semisolid media

are generally used as the basis of to prepare enriched media; hence, known as basal media.

2. Complex Media

Media that contain some ingredients of unknown chemical composition are called **complex media**.

Nutrient Broth

A commonly used complex medium, **nutrient broth (in liquid form)**. It is a simple basal liquid medium, supports growth of many organisms.

Nutrient Agar (Table 7.1)

Nutrient agar is prepared by adding agar at a concentration of 2% to the nutrient broth.

3. Synthetic or Chemically Defined Media

They are prepared exclusively from pure chemical substances and their exact composition is known.

TABLE 7.1: Representative types of agar media.

Medium	Composition	Characteristics
A. Simple medium		
Nutrient agar	Nutrient broth, agar (2–3%)	Complex medium used for routine laboratory work
B. Enriched media		
i. Blood agar	Nutrient agar. Sheep blood (5–10%)	In addition to being enriched medium, it is an indicator medium showing the hemolytic properties of bacteria such as *Streptococcus* pyogenes
ii. Chocolate agar	Heated blood agar (55°C × 2 hours)	Culture fastidious of *Haemophilus influenzae, Neisseria* and *Pnemococcus*
iii. Loeffler's serum slope (LSS)	❖ Nutrient broth ❖ Serum (of ox, sheep or horse) ❖ Glucose	Culture of *Corynebacterium diphtheriae*
C. Indicator media		
MacConkey agar	❖ Peptone ❖ Sodium taurocholate ❖ Agar ❖ Neutral red ❖ Lactose	Isolation and differentiation of lactose fermenting (LF) and nonlactose fermenting (NLF) enteric bacilli
D. Selective media		
Deoxycholate citrate agar (DCA)	❖ Nutrient agar ❖ Sodium deoxycholate ❖ Sodium citrate ❖ Lactose ❖ Neutral red	Suitable for the isolation of *Salmonella* and *Shigella*

C. Special Media (Box 7.1)

1. Enriched Media (Table 7.1)

These are prepared to meet the nutritional requirements of more exacting bacteria by the addition of substances such as blood, serum or egg to a basal medium.

Examples:

i. **Blood agar:** Many medically important bacteria are fastidious, requiring a medium and commonly used in clinical laboratories is **blood agar**.

ii. **Chocolate agar**
iii. **Loeffler's serum slope:** It is used for the isolation of *Corynebacterium diphtheriae*.

2. Enrichment Media (Table 7.2)

When a substance is added to a liquid medium which inhibits the growth of unwanted bacteria and favors the growth of wanted bacteria is known as **enrichment medium**. This medium for an enrichment culture is **usually liquid**.

Usually, the nonpathogenic or commensal bacteria tend to overgrow the pathogenic ones, for example, *Salmonella* (*S*). Typhi being overgrown by *E. coli* in cultures from feces. In such situations, substances which have a stimulating effect on the bacteria to be grown or an inhibitory effect on those to be suppressed are incorporated in the medium.

Examples:
a. **Tetrathionate broth:** Tetrathionate inhibits coliforms while allowing typhoid-paratyphoid bacilli to grow freely in fecal sample.
b. **Selenite F (F for Feces) broth:** It is used for dysentery bacilli.
c. **Alkaline peptone water:** It is used for *Vibrio cholerae* from feces.

3. Selective Media (Table 7.1)

When a substance is added to a solid medium which inhibits the growth of unwanted bacteria but favors the growth of wanted bacteria it is known as **selective media**. These media are used to isolate particular bacteria from specimens where mixed bacterial flora is expected.

Examples of Selective Media:
a. **Deoxycholate citrate agar (DCA):** Addition of deoxycholate acts as a selective agent for dysentery bacilli (isolation of *Shigellae*).
b. **Lowenstein and Jensen medium:** Is used for *Mycobacterium tuberculosis*.
c. **Potassium tellurite medium:** For the isolation of diphtheria bacilli.

TABLE 7.2: Representative types of liquid media.

Medium	Composition	Characteristics
1. Peptone water	❖ Peptone—10 g ❖ Sodium chloride (NaCl)—5 g ❖ Water—1 liter (pH 7.4–7.5)	❖ Basis for carbohydrate fermentation media ❖ For testing the formation of indole
2. Nutrient broth	❖ Peptone water ❖ Meat extract	For routine culture
3. Glucose broth	Nutrient broth + glucose (1% most common)	❖ Blood culture ❖ Promotes luxuriant growth of many organisms ❖ Glucose acts as reducing agent
4. Enrichment media i. Tetrathionate broth	❖ Nutrient broth ❖ Sodium thiosulfate ❖ Calcium carbonate ❖ Iodine solution ❖ Phenol red	Enriches salmonellae and sometimes shigellae
ii. Selenite F broth	❖ Sodium selenite ❖ Peptone ❖ Lactose	It inhibits coliform bacilli while permitting salmonellae and many shigellae to grow
iii. Alkaline peptone water	❖ Peptone—10 g ❖ Sodium chloride (NaCl)—10 g ❖ Distilled water—1 liter	For enriching *V. cholerae* and other *Vibrio* species in a fecal specimen
5. Anaerobic media		
Robertson's cooked meat broth (RCM)	❖ Nutrient broth ❖ Predigested cooked meat of ox heart	❖ Culture of anaerobic bacteria ❖ Preservation of stock culture of aerobic bacteria

4. Indicator Media (Table 7.1)

These media contain an indicator which changes color when a bacterium grows in them.

Example:

a. **MacConkey agar:** MacConkey agar indicates fermenting properties. Lactose fermenter (LF) produce pink colonies and

non-lactose fermenter (NLF) produce colorless colonies due to neutral red indicator.
b. **Wilson and Blair medium:** There is incorporation of sulfite in Wilson and Blair medium. *S. typhi* reduces sulfite to sulfide in the presence of glucose and the colonies of *S. typhi* have a black metallic sheen.

5. Differential Media

A medium which has substances incorporated in it, enabling it to bring out differing characteristics of bacteria and thus helping to distinguish between them, is called a **differential medium. Examples:**
a. **Blood agar**
b. **MacConkey agar:** It is both differential and selective.

6. Sugar Media

For the identification of most of the organisms, sugar fermentation reactions are carried out.

7. Transport Media

A transport medium is a holding medium designed to preserve the viability of microorganisms in the specimen but not allow multiplication.

Delicate organisms (like gonococci) which may not survive the time taken for transporting the specimen to the laboratory or the normal flora may overgrow pathogenic flora *(Salmonella, Shigella* and *V. cholerae)*, such special media are devised to maintain the viability of the pathogen termed as "transport media".

Example: *Stuart's transport medium and Amies transport medium for gonococci.*

D. Anaerobic Media (Table 7.2)

These media are used to grow anaerobic organisms, and contain reducing substances. These include:
  i. Thioglycolate broth
 ii. Cooked meat broth

■ CULTURE METHODS

Methods of Bacterial Culture

The methods of bacterial culture used in the clinical laboratory include **streak culture, lawn culture, stroke culture, stab culture, pour-plate culture, shake culture, and liquid culture.** Special methods are employed for culturing **anaerobic bacteria**.

Streak Culture (Surface Plating)

This method is routinely employed for the isolation of bacteria in pure culture from clinical specimens. A platinum loop No. 23 SWG, 6.5 cm long, is charged with the specimen to be cultured. Owing to the high cost of platinum, loops for routine work are made of nichrome resistance wire, No. 24 SWG. The loop is flat, circular and completely closed with 2–4 mm internal diameter mounted on a handle.

One loopful of the specimen is smeared thoroughly over area A **(Fig. 7.1),** on the surface of a well dried plate, to give a **well-inoculum or "well"**. The loop is resterilized and drawn from the well in two or three parallel lines on to the fresh surface of the medium (B). This process is repeated as shown (C, D, E), care being taken to sterilize the loop, and cool it on unseeded medium, between each sequence. At each step the inoculum is derived from the most distal part of the immediately preceding strokes.

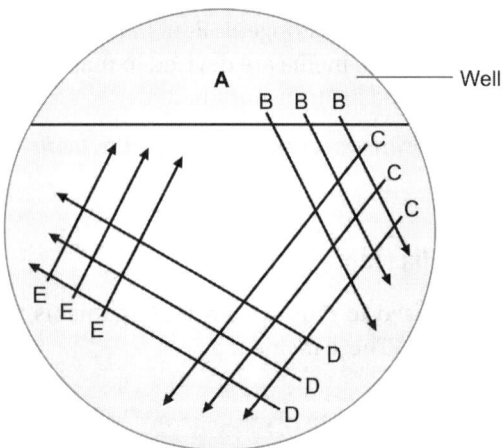

Fig. 7.1: Streak culture (streak plating) on solid media.

Plates are incubated in the inverted position with the lid underneath. On incubation, growth may be confluent at the site of original inoculation ("well"), but becomes progressively thinner, and well separated colonies are obtained over the final series of streaks.

Lawn Culture or Carpet Culture

Lawn cultures are prepared by flooding the surface of the plate with a liquid culture or suspension of the bacterium, pipetting off the excess inoculum and incubating the plate. Alternatively, the surface of the plate may be inoculated by applying a swab soaked in the bacterial culture or suspension. After incubation, lawn culture provides a uniform growth of the bacterium.

Uses
i. Antibiotic susceptibility testing
ii. Bacteriophage typing
iii. For preparation of bacterial antigens and vaccines

Anaerobic Culture Methods

Anaerobic bacteria require incubation without oxygen and differ in their requirement and sensitivity to oxygen. Obligate anaerobes will not grow from small inocula unless oxygen is absent and the pH of the medium is low.

Methods of Anaerobiosis

Anaerobiosis can be achieved by a number of methods.

McIntosh and Fildes anaerobic jar: Anaerobiosis obtained by **McIntosh and Fildes anaerobic jar (Fig. 7.2)** is the most dependable and widely used method.

The jar (20 × 12.5 cm) should be made of metal or robust plastic with a lid that can be clamped down on a gasket to make it airtight. The lid is furnished with two tubes with valves, one acting as gas inlet and the other as the outlet. The lid also has two terminals which can be connected to an electrical supply. On its undersurface it carries a gauze sachet carrying alumina pellets coated with palladium (palladinized alumina). It acts as a room temperature catalyst for the conversion of hydrogen and oxygen into water.

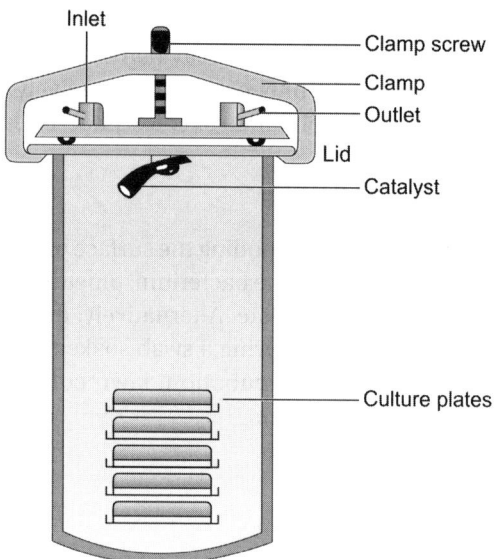

Fig. 7.2: McIntosh and Fildes anaerobic jar.

Procedure: Inoculated culture plates are placed inside the jar with the medium uppermost and lid downward and the lid clamped tight. The outlet tube is connected to a vacuum pump and the air inside is evacuated. Approximately, 6/7 of the air is evacuated (pressure reduced to 100 mm Hg, i.e., 660 mm below atmospheric) and this is monitored on a vacuum gauge. The outlet tap is then closed and the inlet tube connected to a hydrogen supply. Hydrogen is drawn in rapidly.

Catalyst: After the jar is filled with hydrogen, the electrical terminals are connected to a current supply to heat the catalyst and if room temperature catalyst is used, heating is not required. The catalyst will help to combine hydrogen and residual oxygen to form water. The jar is then incubated at 37°C.

Indicator: Reduced methylene blue is generally used as indicator (mixture of NaOH, methylene blue, and glucose). It becomes colorless anaerobically but regains blue color on exposure to oxygen.

By Reducing Agents

Liquid media soon become aerobic unless a reducing agent is added such as glucose, ascorbic acid, cysteine sodium mercaptoacetate or thioglycollate, or the particles of meat in cooked meat broth.

KEY POINTS

A culture medium is any material prepared for the growth of bacteria in a laboratory.
- **Enriched media** are solid media supplemented with blood, serum, etc.
- **Enrichment media:** An enrichment culture is used to encourage the growth of a particular microorganism in a mixed culture and it is the liquid media.
- **Selective media:** By inhibiting unwanted organisms with salts, dyes, or other chemicals, selective media allow growth of only the desired microbes.
- **Transport media** are used to maintain the viability of certain delicate organisms during their transport to the laboratory.
- **Anaerobic jars:** Anaerobiosis obtained by **McIntosh and Fildes anaerobic jar** is the most dependable and widely used method.

IMPORTANT QUESTIONS

1. What are culture media? Classify and discuss them briefly.
2. Distinguish between a selective medium and a differential medium.
3. Discuss anaerobic culture methods in detail.
4. Write short notes on:
    a. Enriched media
    b. Enrichment media
    c. Selective media
    d. Indicator media
    e. Differential media
    f. Transport media
    g. Streak culture
    h. Lawn culture

MULTIPLE CHOICE QUESTIONS (MCQs)

1. The important source of nutrition for bacteria to grow is:
    a. Agar
    b. Electrolytes
    c. Inorganic salts
    d. Peptone

2. All of the following are examples of enriched media, ***except***:
   a. Blood agar
   b. Chocolate agar
   c. Loeffler's serum slope
   d. Bile salt agar
3. All of the following are examples of selective media, ***except***:
   a. Potassium tellurite medium
   b. Deoxycholate citrate agar
   c. Lowenstein and Jensen medium
   d. Nutrient agar
4. Which enrichment medium is preferred to grow ***Vibrio cholerae***?
   a. Tetrathionate broth
   b. Selenite F broth
   c. Alkaline peptone water
   d. All of the above

ANSWERS
1. d   2. d   3. d   4. c

SECTION 3

Infection and its Transmission

Section Outline

- ❖ Infection and Asepsis
- ❖ Collection of Specimens

CHAPTER 8

Infection and Asepsis

Learning Objectives

After reading and studying this chapter, you should be able to:
- Define the terms saprophytes, parasite, commensal, pathogen.
- Describe classification of infections.
- Define and differentiate primary, secondary, opportunistic and reinfections.
- Describe sources of infection giving suitable examples.
- Discuss modes of spread of infection giving suitable examples.
- List the differences between exotoxins and endotoxins.

■ INTRODUCTION

Infection and immunity involve interaction between the animal body (host) and the infecting microorganisms.

Microorganisms and Host

Based on their relationship to their host they can be divided into saprophytes and parasites.

A. **Saprophytes:** Saprophytes (from Greek *sapros* decayed; and *phyton* plant) are free-living microbes that live on dead or decaying organic matter.
B. **Parasites:** Parasites are microbes that can establish themselves and multiply in the hosts. Parasite microbes may be either pathogens or commensals:
   1. **Pathogens:** Pathogens (from Greek *pathos*, disease, and *gen*, to produce) are the microorganisms or agents, which are capable of producing diseases in the host. Its ability to cause disease is called *pathogenicity*.

Types of pathogens
They are two types: **primary** and **opportunist pathogens**.
   a. **Primary (frank) pathogens:** Primary pathogens are the organisms, which are capable of producing disease in previously healthy individuals with intact immunological defenses.
   b. **Opportunist pathogens: Opportunist pathogens** rarely cause disease in individuals with intact immunological and anatomical defenses.
2. **Commensals:** Commensals (organisms of normal flora) are the microorganisms that live in complete harmony with the host without causing any damage to it. Skin and mucous membranes are sterile at birth.

Infection and Infectious Disease

Infection: The lodgment and multiplication of a parasite in or on the tissues of a host constitute **infection.**

Infectious disease: An **infectious disease** is any change from a state of health in which part or all of the host body is not capable of carrying on its normal functions due to the presence of an organism or its products. A clinically manifest disease of man or animals resulting from an infection.

Chain of Infection

For a microorganism to be transported and be effective in continuing contamination, it follows a definite cycle or chain of events. The following **six elements** are necessary for infection to occur **(Fig. 8.1)**:
1. **The infectious agent**—a pathogen
2. **Reservoir:** Any natural habitat of a microorganism that promotes growth and reproduction is a **reservoir.** Examples of reservoirs are soiled or wet dressings and hospital equipment such as a bedside stand, an overbed table, suction equipment, or urinary drainage bags. A **carrier,** or vector, is a person or animal that does not become ill but harbors and spreads an organism, causing disease in others.
3. **Exit route:** A microorganism does not have the capacity to cause disease in another host without finding a point of escape from the reservoir. Successful microbes must leave the body and then be transmitted to fresh hosts. Exit routes in humans are the

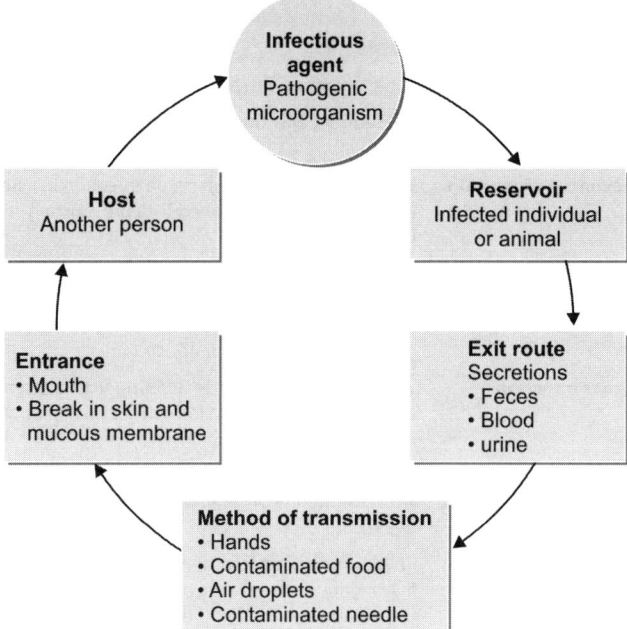

Fig. 8.1: The chain of infection.

gastrointestinal, respiratory, and genitourinary systems; tissue; blood; and wounds.
4. **Method or vehicle of transportation**, such as exudate, feces, air droplets, hands, and needles.
5. **Entrance through skin, mucous lining, or mouth**
6. **Host:** Another person or animal where organism is nourished and harbored.

Prevention

To prevent the spread of a microorganism, the cycle must be interrupted. This is possible through daily practices of medical asepsis. These practices help to inhibit (to stop or slow a process) the growth and reduce the number of microorganisms.

Classification of Infections

Infections may be classified in various ways **(Table 8.1)**.
1. **Primary infection:** Initial infection with a parasite in a host is termed *primary infection.*

TABLE 8.1: Classification of infections.

Infection	Details
1. Primary infection	Initial infection with a parasite in a host
2. Reinfections	Subsequent infections by the same parasite in the host
3. Secondary infection	When a new parasite sets up an infection in a host whose resistance is lowered by a pre-existing infectious disease
4. Local infection	The term *Local infection* (more appropriately *local sepsis*) indicates a condition where, due to infection or sepsis at localized sites such as appendix or tonsils, generalized effects are produced
5. Cross infection	When in a patient already suffering from a disease a new infection is set up from other host or another external source
6. Healthcare-associated infections (HAIs)	**HAIs** include those with hospital onset and those with community onset in patients with previous healthcare encounters
7. Iatrogenic infection	Physician induced infections resulting from investigative, therapeutic or other procedures. Depending on whether the source of infection is from the host's own body or from external sources, infections are classified as *endogenous* or *exogenous*, respectively
8. Inapparent infection	Inapparent infection is one where clinical effects are not apparent
9. Subclinical infection	The term *subclinical infection* is often used as a synonym to inapparent infection
10. Atypical infection	Atypical infection is one in which the typical or characteristic clinical manifestations of the particular infectious disease are not present
11. Latent infection	Some parasites, following infection, may remain in the tissues in a latent or hidden form proliferating and producing clinical disease when the host resistance is lowered. This is termed *latent infection*

2. **Reinfections:** Subsequent infections by the same parasite in the host are termed *reinfections*.
3. **Secondary infection:** When a new parasite sets up an infection in a host whose resistance is lowered by a pre-existing infectious disease, this is termed *secondary infection*.
4. **Local infection:** The term *local infection* (more appropriately *local sepsis*) indicates a condition where, due to infection or sepsis

at localized sites, such as appendix or tonsils, generalized effects are produced.
5. **Cross infection:** When in a patient already suffering from a disease, a new infection is set up from other host or another external source, it is termed *cross infection*.
6. **Nosocomial infections:** Cross infections occurring in hospitals are called *nosocomial infections* (from Greek *nosocomial* hospital).
7. **Iatrogenic infection:** The term *iatrogenic infection* refers to physician-induced infections resulting from investigative, therapeutic, or other procedures. Based on the clinical effects of infections, they may be classified into different varieties.
8. **Inapparent infection:** Inapparent infection is one where clinical effects are not apparent.
9. **Subclinical infection:** The term *subclinical infection* is often used as a synonym to inapparent infection.
10. **Atypical infection:** Atypical infection is one in which the typical or characteristic clinical manifestations of the particular infectious disease are not present.
11. **Latent infection:** Some parasites, following infection, may remain in the tissues in a latent or hidden form proliferating and producing clinical disease when the host resistance is lowered. This is termed *latent infection*.

Sources of Infection

A. **Human beings:** The most common source of infection for human beings is human beings themselves. The parasite may originate from a patient or carrier. Humans play a substantial role as microbial reservoirs.
   Carrier: A **carrier** is person who harbors the microorganisms without suffering from any ill effect because of it. There are several types of carriers.
B. **Animals:**
   - **Reservoir hosts:** Many pathogens are capable of causing infections in both human beings and animals. Therefore, animals may act as a source of infection of such organisms. These, animals serve to maintain the parasite in nature and act as **reservoir** and they are, therefore, called **reservoir hosts**.
   - **Zoonosis:** The diseases and infections, which are transmissible to man from animals, are called **zoonosis**. Humans contract the pathogens by several mechanisms.

Examples of zoonotic diseases:
- **Bacterial:** Anthrax, brucellosis, Q fever, leptospirosis, bovine tuberculosis, bubonic plague, Salmonella food poisoning.
- **Viral:** Rabies, yellow fever, cowpox, monkeypox.
- **Protozoal:** Leishmaniasis, toxoplasmosis, trypanosomiasis, babesiosis.
- **Helminthic:** Echinococcosis, taeniasis, trichinellosis.
- **Fungal:** *Microsporum canis, trichophyton verrucosum.*

C. **Insects:**
- **Arthropod-borne diseases:** Blood-sucking insects such as mosquitoes, ticks, mites, flies, and lice may transmit pathogens to human beings and diseases, so caused are called *arthropod borne diseases.*
- **Vectors:** Insects that transmit infections are called *vectors.*
- **Reservoir hosts:** Besides acting as vectors, some insects may also act as reservoir hosts (e.g., ticks in relapsing fever and spotted fever). Infection is maintained in such insects by transovarial or transstadial passage.

D. **Soil and water:**
  i. **Soil:** Some pathogens can survive in the soil for long periods. **Examples: (a) Spores of tetanus and gas gangrene (b) Fungi and parasites**.
  ii. Water

E. **Food**

Modes of Transmission of Infection

Pathogenic organisms can spread from one host to another by a variety of mechanisms. These include:

1. **Contact:** Infection may be acquired by contact, which may be direct or indirect.
   a. **Direct contact:** Such as sexually transmitted diseases.
   b. **Indirect contact:** Indirect contact may be through the agency of fomites, which are inanimate objects, such as clothing, pencils or toys, which may be contaminated by a pathogen from one person and act as a vehicle for its transmission to another.
2. **Inhalation:** Respiratory infections such as common cold, influenza, measles, mumps, tuberculosis and whooping cough are acquired by inhalation.

3. **Ingestion:** Intestinal infections are generally acquired by the ingestion of food or drink contaminated by pathogens. Infection transmitted by ingestion may be waterborne (cholera), food borne (food poisoning), or handborne (dysentery).
4. **Inoculation:** The disease agent may be inoculated directly into the skin or mucosa, e.g., rabies virus deposited subcutaneously by dog bite, tetanus spores implanted in deep wounds, and arboviruses is injected by insect vectors. Infection by inoculation may be iatrogenic when unsterile syringes and surgical equipment are employed, e.g., hepatitis B and the human immunodeficiency virus (HIV).
5. **Insects (see under sources of infection):** *Vector* is defined as an arthropod or any living carrier (e.g., snail) that transports an infectious agent to a susceptible individual.
6. **Congenital:** Some pathogens are able to cross the placental barrier and reach the fetus in utero. This is known as **vertical transmission**. **Examples:** So-called TORCH *(Toxoplasma gondii,* rubella virus, cytomegalovirus, and herpes virus) agents, varicella virus, syphilis, hepatitis B, coxsackie B and acquired immunodeficiency syndrome (AIDS).
7. **Iatrogenic and laboratory infections:** If meticulous care in asepsis is not taken, infections like AIDS and hepatitis B may sometimes be transmitted during administration of injections, lumbar puncture, and catheterization.

■ FACTORS PREDISPOSING TO MICROBIAL PATHOGENICITY

Pathogenicity and Virulence

Pathogenicity denotes the ability of a microbial species to cause disease. The term virulence (Latin *virulentia,* from *virus,* poison) denotes the ability of a strain of a species to produce disease.

Virulence provides a quantitative measure of pathogenicity, or the likelihood of causing disease.

Determinants of Virulence

1. **Transmissibility:** The first step of the infectious process is the entry of the microorganism into the host by one of several ports: the respiratory tract, gastrointestinal tract, urogenital tract, or through skin that has been cut, punctured, or burned.

2. **Adhesion:** The initial event in the pathogenesis is the attachment of the bacteria to body surfaces.
3. **Invasiveness:** Invasiveness signifies the ability of a pathogen to spread in the host tissues after establishing infection. For many disease-producing bacteria, invasion of the host's epithelium is central to the infectious process. Highly invasive pathogens characteristically produce spreading or generalized lesions (e.g., streptococcal septicemia following wound infection), while less invasive pathogens cause more localized lesions (e.g., staphylococcal abscess).
4. **Toxigenicity:** Some bacteria cause disease by producing toxins, of which there are two general types: the exotoxins and the endotoxins **(Table 8.2)**.
   a. **Exotoxins:** These are soluble, heat-labile proteins inactivated at 60–80°C which are secreted by certain species of bacteria and diffuse readily into the surrounding medium.
   b. **Endotoxins:** These are heat-stable, lipopolysaccharide (LPS) components of the outer membranes of gram-negative but not gram-positive bacteria. Their toxicity depends upon the component (lipid A). Intravenous injections of large doses of endotoxin and massive gram-negative septicemias cause endotoxic shock **(Table 8.2)**.
5. **Avoidance of host-defense mechanisms:** Bacteria also have evolved many mechanisms to evade host defenses. Several of these evasive mechanisms are such as **capsules**.
6. **Enzymes:** Many species of bacteria produce tissue-degrading enzymes that play important roles in the infection process.
   i. *Coagulase:* Coagulase is produced by *S. aureus* and prevents phagocytosis.
   ii. *Hyaluronidase:* Hyaluronidase facilitates the spread of infection along tissue spaces.
7. **Plasmids:** Plasmids are extra chromosomal DNA segments that carry genes for antibiotic resistance known as R-factors. Multiple drug resistance (R) plasmids increase the severity of clinical disease by their resistance to antibiotic therapy.
8. **Bacteriophages:** The classical example of phage-directed virulence is seen in diphtheria.
9. **Communicability:** The ability of a microbe to spread from one host to another is known as communicability.

TABLE 8.2: Differences between exotoxins and endotoxins.

Exotoxins	Endotoxins
❖ Proteins	❖ Lipopolysaccharide on outer membrane. Lipid A portion is toxic
❖ Heat-labile (inactivated at 60–80°C)	❖ Heat-stable
❖ Actively secreted by the cells; diffuse into the surrounding medium	❖ Form integral part of the cell wall; do not diffuse into surrounding medium
❖ Readily separable from cultures by physical means such as filtration	❖ Obtained only by cell lysis
❖ Action often enzymic	❖ No enzymic action
❖ Specific pharmacological effect for each exotoxin	❖ Nonspecific action of all endotoxins
❖ Specific tissue affinities	❖ No specific tissue affinities
❖ Highly toxic and fatal in microgram quantities	❖ Moderate toxicity. Active only in very large doses
❖ Highly antigenic	❖ Weakly antigenic
❖ Action specifically neutralized by antibody	❖ Neutralization by antibody ineffective
❖ Usually do not produce fever	❖ Usually produce fever by release of interlukin-1
❖ Produced by both gram-positive bacteria and gram-negative bacteria	❖ Produced by gram-negative bacteria only
❖ Frequently controlled by extrachromosomal genes (e.g., plasmids)	❖ Synthesized directly by chromosomal genes
❖ Examples: Botulism diphtheria tetanus	❖ Examples: Gram-negative infections, meningococcemia

10. **Infecting dose:** Adequate number of bacteria is required for successful infections. The dosage may be estimated as the *minimum infecting dose* (MID) or *minimum lethal dose* (MLD).
11. **Route of infection:** Certain bacteria are infective when introduced through optimal route, for example, *Vibrio cholerae* can produce lesion only when administered by oral route, but unable to cause infection when introduced subcutaneously.

Types of Infectious Diseases

Infectious diseases may be localized or generalized.
A. **Localized:** Localized infections may be superficial or deep seated.
B. **Generalized:** Bacteremia, septicemia, and pyemia.

ASEPSIS

Asepsis is absence of pathogenic microorganisms. It is divided into two categories: (1) medical and (2) surgical.
1. **Medical asepsis (clean technique):** It consists of techniques that inhibit the growth and spread of pathogenic microorganisms. Medical asepsis is also known as **clean technique** and is used in many daily activities. They include hand washing, bathing, cleaning environment, gloving, gowning, wearing masks, hair and shoe covers, disinfecting articles, and use of antiseptics changing patients' bed linen. You follow principles of medical asepsis in the home, for instance, with the common practice of washing your hands before preparing food.
2. **Surgical asepsis (sterile technique):** It destroys all microorganisms and their **spores** (the reproductive cell of some microorganisms, such as fungi or protozoa). Surgical asepsis is known as **sterile technique** and is used in specialized areas or skills, such as care of surgical wounds, urinary catheter insertion, invasive procedures, and surgery.

Healthcare-associated Infections

Healthcare-associated infections (HAIs) include those with hospital onset and community onset in patients with previous healthcare encounters.
- **Sources of infections:**
  A. **Exogenous:** Exogenous source may be another person in the hospital *(cross-infection)* or a contaminated item of equipment or building service *(environmental infection).*
  B. **Endogenous:** The infecting organisms are derived from the patient's own skin, gastrointestinal, or upper respiratory flora.

Types of **healthcare-associated infections:**
1. Catheter-associated urinary tract infections (CAUTI)
2. Ventilator-associated pneumonia (VAP)
3. Central line-associated bloodstream infection (CLABSI)
4. Surgical site infections (SSIs)

Diagnosis and control of hospital infection: The most important steps in preventing nosocomial infections are to first recognize their occurrence and then establish policies to prevent their development. Hospital infection may occur sporadically or as outbreaks.

Infection Control Policy

There will normally be two parts:
1. **Infection control committee (ICC)**
2. **Infection control team**

Prevention of hospital associated infections:
1. Standard/universal precautions
2. Precautions for prevention of transmission of infection
3. **Bundles in infection:** Care "bundles" are simple sets of evidence-based practices that, when implemented collectively, improve the reliability of their delivery and improve patient outcomes. **Specific care bundles** include bundles for the prevention of CLABSI, bundle for the prevention of CAUTI, bundle for the prevention of VAP, and bundle for the prevention of SSI.

Defenses Against Infection

- Natural barriers and the immune system defend the body against organisms that can cause infection.
- Natural barriers include the skin, mucous membranes, tears, earwax, mucus, and stomach acid. Also, the normal flow of urine washes out microorganisms that enter the urinary tract.
- The immune system uses white blood cells and antibodies to identify and eliminate organisms that get through the body's natural barriers. **(For details *see* Chapter 10: Immunity).**

KEY POINTS

- Parasites are microbes that can establish themselves and multiply in the hosts. Parasite microbes may be either pathogens or commensals.
- **Sources of infection: (A) Human beings, (B) Animals, (C) Insects, (D) Soil and water, (E) Food**
- **Modes of transmission of infection: (1) Contact, (2) Inhalation, (3) Ingestion, (4) Inoculation, (5) Insects, (6) Congenital, (7) Iatrogenic and laboratory infections.**
- Pathogenicity denotes the ability of a microbial species to cause disease. The term virulence denotes the ability of a strain of a species to produce disease. Enhancement of virulence is known as *exaltation*. Reduction of virulence is known as *attenuation*.

Section 3: Infection and its Transmission

IMPORTANT QUESTIONS
1. Describe in detail the sources of infections to human beings.
2. What are the various modes of spread of infection? Describe each in brief giving suitable examples.
3. Distinguish between exotoxins and endotoxins in a tabulated form.

MULTIPLE CHOICE QUESTIONS (MCQs)
1. The organisms can be transmitted vertically by all the following ways, except:
    a. Sexual contact
    b. Through the placenta
    c. Within the birth canal
    d. Through breast milk
2. Which of the following may cause teratogenic infections?
    a. Toxoplasma
    b. Rubella virus
    c. Cytomegalovirus
    d. All of the above
3. Which of the following statement is not true for exotoxins?
    a. They are proteins
    b. They are highly antigenic
    c. They are heat-labile
    d. They are obtained by cell lysis
4. Which of the statement is not true for endotoxins?
    a. These are lipopolysaccharides component of outer membrane of gram-negative bacteria
    b. These are heat-stable
    c. They cannot be toxoid
    d. They are highly antigenic
5. The disease that spreads rapidly, involving many persons in a particular area at the same time is known as:
    a. Sporadic
    b. Endemic
    c. Epidemic
    d. Pandemic

ANSWERS
1. a   2. d   3. d   4. d   5. c

CHAPTER 9

Collection of Specimens

Learning Objectives

After reading and studying this chapter, you should be able to:
- Describe universal precautions.
- Describe procedures used for taking clinical specimens from a patient with various infectious diseases.
- Discuss identification of microorganisms from specimens.

■ INTRODUCTION

Diagnostic medical microbiology is concerned with the etiologic diagnosis of infection. Once isolated and identified, the microorganism can then be subjected to antimicrobial sensitivity tests. Computers and advances in technology for rapid identification, some commercially available, have greatly aided the clinical microbiologist.

■ SPECIMENS

In clinical microbiology, a clinical specimen (hereafter, specimen) represents a portion or quantity of human material that is, tested, examined, or studied to determine the presence or absence of particular microorganisms. Samples for microbiological examination need to be carefully collected, if possible without contamination with commensals or from external sources. It is essential to use sterile containers, which are leak-proof and able to withstand transportation through the post, if necessary. Special precautions required for "high-risk" specimens need to be defined by the laboratory and hospital management.

Other important concerns regarding specimens:
1. The specimen selected should adequately represent the diseased area and also may include additional sites (e.g., liver and blood

specimens) in order to isolate and identify potential agents of the particular disease process.
2. A quantity of specimen adequate in amount to allow a variety of diagnostic testing should be obtained.
3. Attention must be given to specimen collection in order to avoid contamination from the different varieties of microorganisms indigenous to the skin and mucous membrane.
4. The specimen should be forwarded promptly to the clinical laboratory.
5. If possible, the specimen should be obtained before antimicrobial agents have been administered to the patient.

■ UNIVERSAL PRECAUTIONS

Concerns about transmission of the hepatitis B virus (HBV) and human immunodeficiency virus (HIV) led to the introduction of "universal precautions", to minimize the infections in medical laboratory workers and healthcare personnel. These universal precautions include:
1. Assume that all specimens/patients are potentially infectious for HIV and other blood-borne pathogens.
2. All blood specimens or body fluids should be placed in a leak-proof impervious bag for transportation to the laboratory.
3. Use gloves while handling blood and body fluid specimens and other objects exposed to them. If there is a likelihood of spattering, use face masks with glasses or goggles.
4. Wear laboratory coats or gowns while working in the laboratory. Wrap-around gowns should be preferred. These should not be taken outside.
5. Never pipette by mouth. Mechanical pipetting devices should be used.
6. Decontaminate the laboratory work surfaces with an appropriate disinfectant after the spillage of blood or other body fluids and when the procedures are completed.
7. Limit use of needles and syringes to situations for which there are no other alternatives.
8. Biological safety hoods should be used for laboratory work.

■ COLLECTION

Specimens may be collected by several methods using aseptic technique:

Infections of Wounds and Other Tissues

Pus or *exudate* is often submitted on a swab for laboratory investigation. Whenever possible, pus or exudate should be submitted in a small screw-capped bottle, a firmly stoppered tube or syringe, or a sealed capillary tube. Fragments of excised tissue removed at wound toilet, or curettings from infected sinuses and other tissues, should be sent in a sterile container without fixative.

Upper Respiratory, Ear, and Eye Infections

1. An adequate view of the throat should be ensured by good lighting and the use of a disposable wooden spatula to pull outward and so depress the tongue.
2. **Oral cavity:** The most common method used to collect specimens from the anterior nares or throat is the sterile swab.
   Anterior nares: If pus is present, collect this on swabs. If no pus is present, moisten swabs and then swab the anterior nares.
   Throat for bacteriological sampling: A plain, albumen-coated, or charcoal-coated cotton-wool swab should be used to collect as much exudate as possible from the tonsils, posterior pharyngeal wall and any other area that is inflamed or bears exudate. The swab should be replaced in its tube with care not to soil the rim. If it cannot be delivered to the laboratory within about 1 hour, it should be placed in a refrigerator at 4°C until delivery or, preferably, it should be submitted in a tube of transport medium for bacteriological specimens.
3. **Nasopharyngeal swabs:**
   Pernasal swab: Collection of nasopharyngeal secretion by a *pernasal* swab in charcoal transport medium for the diagnosis of whooping cough.
   Postnasal swab: A postnasal swab may be used for the detection of potential pathogens carried in the nasopharynx of healthy persons, e.g., *Meningococcus*.
4. **The glottis and epiglottis:** Swabs are firmly rubbed over inflamed and ulcerated areas.
5. **Paranasal sinuses:** If pus is present in these sinuses, it is collected on swabs or aspirated with a syringe and needle.

Gastrointestinal Tract

Feces and rectal swabs are the most readily available specimens.
1. **Feces:** Feces are collected in a container, which is a 25 mL screw-capped, wide-mouthed, glass or plastic bottle.

2. **Fresh feces** may be collected by inserting well and twisted around several times a soft-rubber catheter into the rectum. Transmit the specimen quickly to the laboratory.
3. **In suspected parasitic infestations:** For examination for parasites, a small sample may be taken from a morning stool microscopic examination for eggs and adult parasites. The sample is placed in a preservative (polyvinyl alcohol, buffered glycerol, saline, or formalin) for microscopic examination for eggs and adult parasites.

From the Lower Respiratory Tract

Sputum: Sputum is the most common specimen collected in suspected cases of lower respiratory tract infections. A morning sample is best. Sputum is collected in especially designed sputum cups.

Stomach aspiration: In cases such as tuberculosis in which there is little sputum, stomach aspiration may be necessary.

Urinary Tract Infections

After the patient has cleansed the urethral meatus (opening), a small container is used to collect the urine. Instruct the patient to collect a **midstream sample.** A urine sample may be stored under refrigeration (4–6°C) for up to 24 hours.

From the Genital Tract

1. **Genital infections in women:**
   High vaginal swab: The specimen generally collected for the diagnosis of vaginitis, vaginosis, or uterine sepsis.
2. **In** suspected infections due to *Neisseria gonorrhoeae*.
   In women: An *endocervical swab* must be collected for examination for gonococci. **Rectal and pharyngeal swabs** should also be considered. Swabs for culture should be placed in tubes of Amies' transport medium for delivery to the laboratory.
3. **Collection of specimens in men:**
   i. **Urethral discharge:** Urethral discharge milked from the urethra may be expressed directly on to slides for examination in Gram-stained films for gonococci. Discharge collected in an inoculating loop should, if possible, be inoculated immediately on to warmed plates of heated-blood agar and selective

medium for the culture of gonococci. If specimens have to be transported to the laboratory for the preparation of films and inoculation into culture, as much exudate as possible should be collected on a swab and the swab at once plunged into a tube of Amies' transport medium.

    ii. **Massage of the prostate per rectum:** When **prostatitis** is suspected and there is no spontaneous discharge from the urethra, massage of the prostate *per rectum* may express some exudate for examination.

4. **In suspected infections due to *Treponema pallidum*:** The examination of a chancre requires the careful collection of exudate and its preparation for dark ground microscopy. A specimen of clotted venous blood should be collected for serological examination.
5. **In suspected infections due to *Trichomonas*:** For *Trichomonas* examination, further, special specimens should be collected from the vagina and cervix, including a swab placed in clear *Trichomonas* transport medium for microscopy and possibly culture.

From the Central Nervous System

The principle specimen to be examined is of cerebrospinal fluid (CSF) collected by lumbar puncture. Only 3–5 mL of fluid should be collected. The specimen must be dispatched to the laboratory as quickly as possible, for delay may result in the death of delicate pathogens, such as meningococci, and the disintegration of leukocytes. It should not be kept in a refrigerator, which tends to kill *Haemophilus* (*H*) *influenzae*. If delay for a few hours is unavoidable, the specimen is best kept in an incubator at 37°C.

From the Bloodstream

With precautions to avoid touching and recontaminating the venipuncture site, take the sample of blood. Inoculate the required volume into each blood culture bottle.

It is essential to avoid contamination of the sample or the operator. Therefore it is most important to prepare the skin properly before venipuncture for blood culture.

1. The operator's hands must be clean and dry. Sterile gloves may be worn if there is any possibility of a specific hazard such as hepatitis B or HIV. Palpation for the vein can be checked with a gloved finger.

2. Disinfect the venipuncture site on the patient's skin by applying 70% isopropyl alcohol in water with 1% iodine or 1-2% chlorhexidine scrubbed in a concentric fashion around the venipuncture site for at least 1 minute and allow to dry.
3. With precautions to avoid touching and recontaminating the venipuncture site, take the sample of blood.
4. Detach and safely discard the sampling needle. Then fit a fresh sterile needle and inoculate the required volume into each blood culture bottle.
5. After the venipuncture, the disinfecting agent should be removed with an alcohol pad.

From Wound or Abscess

1. Cleanse the area with a sterile swab moistened in sterile saline.
2. Disinfect the area with 70% ethanol or iodine solution.
3. If the abscess has not ruptured spontaneously, a physician will open it with a sterile scalpel.
4. Wipe the first pus away.
5. Touch a sterile swab to the pus, taking care not to contaminate the surrounding tissue.
6. Replace the swab in its container, and properly label the container.
7. Pus, if present in a large amount, should preferably be collected in a bottle.

Fluid from Pleural and Peritoneal Cavities

These cavities and joints are normally sterile. Hence, specimens have to be collected from these sites as carefully as are CSF and blood specimens. These sites may be involved in acute (pyogenic) or in chronic (tuberculous) disease processes.

From the Conjunctiva, Lid Margins, Cornea, and Intraocular Structures

Eye Infections

1. The exudate should be picked up with a sterile platinum loop or on the smoothly rounded tip of a thin glass or plastic rod; otherwise, on the tip of a thin serum-coated swab. It should be collected from the **conjunctiva,** e.g., from under an everted eyelid, and contamination from the skin and margin of the eyelid should be

avoided. A separate collection should be made for inoculation on to each culture plate and for the making of a smear.
2. Material for chlamydia culture should be sent in an appropriate transport medium. Conjunctival swabs for virology should be sent in a virus transport medium, together with a throat swab if adenovirus infection is suspected.
3. If the patient is suffering from a corneal ulcer, material is obtained from the base and edges of the ulcer by using a sterile blade or spatula; this material is at once inoculated onto appropriate bacterial and fungal culture media. Smears are made for staining by various methods.
4. **Infections of orbit and eyeball:** Any exudate obtainable should be examined for such organisms and a blood culture should be done. *Iritis* and *chorioretinitis* may occur in the course of systemic viral infections, e.g., with cytomegalovirus, and also in toxoplasmosis, for which serological diagnosis should be attempted.
5. If the patient is suffering from endophthalmitis or other intraocular lesion, material is aspirated from the vitreous or aqueous humor by a sterile syringe and needle, and processed as appropriate.

Ear Infections

Swabs are taken from the external auditory meatus mainly in three suspected conditions, acute otitis media, chronic suppurative otitis media and otitis externa.

■ TRANSPORT OF SPECIMENS

Speed in transporting the specimen to the clinical laboratory after it has been obtained from the patient is of prime importance. CSF should be examined immediately transported to the laboratory within 15 minutes. Special treatment is required for specimens when the microorganism is thought to be anaerobic. Microbiological specimens may be transported to the laboratory by various means.

■ HEALTH AND SAFETY PRECAUTIONS

Observe universal precautions when collecting specimens.

Follow proper blood collection techniques to minimize the risk of transmitting infectious diseases to clinical staff, and wear gloves when appropriate.

Dispose of syringes and needles in a puncture-resistant, autoclavable discard container. A new sterile syringe and needle must be used for each patient.

For transport to a microbiology laboratory, place the specimen in a container that can be securely sealed.

Remove gloves and discard in an autoclavable container.

Wash hands with antibacterial soap and water immediately after removing gloves.

In the event of a needle-stick injury or other skin puncture or wound, wash the wound liberally with soap and water. Encourage bleeding.

Report a needle-stick injury, any other skin puncture, or any contamination of the hands or body with CSF to the supervisor and appropriate health officials immediately as prophylactic treatment of the personnel performing the procedure may be indicated.

KEY POINT

Collection: Specimens may be collected by several methods using aseptic technique from various infections.

IMPORTANT QUESTIONS

1. How can clinical specimens be taken from a patient with various infectious diseases? Give specific examples of procedures used.
2. Write short notes on:
   a. Universal precautions
   b. Health and safety precautions

MULTIPLE CHOICE QUESTIONS (MCQs)

1. Clinical specimens are collected:
   a. By using sterile containers which are leak-proof
   b. By using aseptic technique
   c. All of the above
   d. None of the above
2. For urinary tract infections:
   a. Collect a midstream sample of urine
   b. No need to cleanse the urethral meatus (opening)
   c. Any container can be used
   d. Never store under refrigeration

ANSWERS

1. c   2. a

SECTION 4

Immunology

Section Outline

- ❖ Immunity
- ❖ Immunoprophylaxis
- ❖ Hypersensitivity Reactions
- ❖ Autoimmunity
- ❖ Principles and Uses of Serological Tests

CHAPTER 10

Immunity

Learning Objectives

After reading and studying this chapter, you should be able to:
- Describe innate immunity, artificial active immunity, natural passive immunity, and herd immunity.
- Differentiate between active and passive immunity.

▪ DEFINITION

Immunity refers to the resistance exhibited by the host toward injury caused by microorganisms and their products.

The complex reaction a host animal undergoes after contact with microorganisms can be grouped under the broadly defined heading of **resistance**.

▪ CLASSIFICATION

Immunity against infectious diseases is of different types. The discrimination between self and nonself, and the subsequent destruction and removal of foreign material, is accomplished by two arms of immune system, the **innate** (or **"natural"**) **immune system**, and the **adaptive** (or **"acquired"**), **specific immune system**.

Innate or Natural Immunity

It is the resistance to infections which an individual possesses by virtue of his genetic or constitutional make up. Repeated exposure to a pathogen does not enhance the innate immune system.

Nonspecific and Specific Immunity

It may be **nonspecific**, when it indicates a degree of resistance to infections in general, or **specific** where resistance to a particular pathogen is concerned. Innate immunity may be considered at the level of **species, race or individual.**

■ MECHANISMS OF INNATE IMMUNITY

1. **Mechanical barriers and surface secretions:**
   A. **Skin:** The intact skin and the mucous membranes provide mechanical barriers. Secretions from the sebaceous glands contain both saturated and unsaturated fatty acids that kill many bacteria and fungi.
   B. **Mucous membrane:**
   General protective mechanisms: A major protective component of mucous membranes is the **mucus** itself.
   Specific protective characteristics:
      i. **Mouth or oral cavity:** The mouth or oral cavity is protected by the flow of saliva that physically carries microorganisms away from the cell surfaces and also contains the lysozyme, which destroys bacterial cell walls, and antibodies.
      ii. **Gastrointestinal tract:** The low pH and proteolytic enzymes of the stomach help to keep the numbers of microorganisms low. In the **small intestine**, protection is provided by the presence of bile salts.
      iii. **Upper respiratory tract:** Cough reflex is an important defense mechanism of the respiratory tract. Nasal and respiratory secretions contain **mucopolysaccharide** capable of combining with influenza and certain other viruses.
      vi. **Genitourinary tract:**
         a. **Normal flow of urine:** The normal flow of urine flushes the urinary system.
         b. **Spermine and zinc:** Spermine and zinc present in the semen carry out antibacterial activity.
         c. **Acidity of the adult vagina:** The low pH (acidity) of the adult vagina provides an inhospitable environment for colonization by pathogens.

v. **Conjunctiva:** Conjunctiva is continually being assaulted by microbe-laden dust and is kept moist by the continuous flushing action of tears (lacrimal fluid). Tears contain the antibacterial substance lysozyme.
2. **Antibacterial substances in blood and tissues:** Many microbial substances are present in the tissue and body fluids. These are nonspecific:
   - Complement system
   - Other substances.
3. **Microbial antagonisms:** The skin and mucous surfaces have resident bacterial flora which prevent colonization by pathogens.
4. **Cellular factors in innate immunity:** Natural defense against the invasion of blood and tissues by microorganisms and other foreign particles is mediated to a large extent by phagocytic cells which ingest and destroy them.
5. **Inflammation:** If the surface chemical and physiologic defenses of the body are breached by a pathogen, inflammation can result, which is an important, nonspecific defense mechanism.
6. **Fever:** Following infection a rise of temperature is a natural defense mechanism.
7. **Acute phase proteins:** A sudden increase in the plasma concentration of certain proteins, collectively termed "**acute phase proteins**" occurs as a result of infection or tissue injury.

■ TYPES OF IMMUNITY

Acquired Immunity

Acquired immunity refers to the resistance that an individual acquires during his lifetime. Acquired immunity is of two types: (1) active immunity, and (2) passive immunity **(Table 10.1)**.

Active Immunity

Active immunity is induced after contact with foreign antigens.

Immune response:

A. **The primary response:** Active immunity sets in only after a **latent period**. There is often a **negative phase**. Once developed, the active immunity is **long lasting**.

TABLE 10.1: Comparison of active and passive immunity.

Active immunity	Passive immunity
Produced actively by host's immune system	Received passively. No active host participation
Induced by infection or by immunogens	Readymade antibody transferred
Durable effective protection	Transient, less effective
Immunity effective only after lag period, i.e., time required for generation of antibodies and immunocompetent cells	Immediate immunity
Immunological memory present	No memory
Booster effect on subsequent dose	Subsequent dose less effective
"Negative phase" may occur	No negative phase
Not applicable in the immunodeficient	Applicable in immunodeficient

B. **Secondary response:** If an individual who has been actively immunized against an antigen, experiences the same antigen subsequently, the immune response occurs more quickly and abundantly than during the first encounter. This is known as **secondary response.**

Types of active immunity:

1. **Natural active immunity:** Natural active immunity results from either a clinical or an inapparent infection by a microbe.
   Such immunity is usually **long lasting**. The immunity is **life-long** following many viral diseases such as chickenpox or measles.
2. **Artificial active immunity:** Artificial active immunity is the resistance induced by vaccines. **Vaccines** are preparations of live or killed microorganisms or their products used for immunization. Vaccines are made with either (1) live, attenuated microorganisms; (2) killed microorganisms; (3) microbial extract; (4) vaccine conjugates; or (5) inactivated toxoids.
   Both bacterial and viral pathogens are targeted by these diverse means.

Examples of Vaccines
1. **Bacterial vaccines**
   a. Live (BCG vaccine for tuberculosis)
   b. Killed (cholera vaccine)
   c. Subunit (typhoid Vi antigen)
   d. Bacterial products (tetanus toxoid)
2. **Viral vaccines**
   a. *Live:*
      - Oral polio vaccine—Sabin
      - 17D vaccine for yellow fever
      - MMR vaccine for measles, mumps, rubella
   b. *Killed:* Injectable polio vaccine—Salk
      - Neural and non-neural vaccines for rabies
      - Hepatitis B vaccine
   c. *Subunit:* Hepatitis B vaccine

Passive Immunity

The immunity that is transferred to a recipient in a "readymade" form is known as **passive immunity**.

Main advantage of passive immunity:

❖ The prompt availability of large amount of antibody.
❖ It is employed where **instant immunity** is required because of its immediate action.

1. Natural Passive Immunity

This is the resistance passively transferred from mother to baby through the placenta. After birth, immunoglobulins (Ig) are passed to the newborn through the **breast milk.** The **human colostrum**, is rich in IgA antibodies, which gives protection to the neonate up to 3 months of age.

2. Artificial Passive Immunity

Artificial passive immunity is the resistance passively transferred to a recipient by the administration of antibodies. The agents used for this purpose are pooled human gamma globulin, hyperimmune sera of animal or human origin and convalescent sera. These are used for prophylaxis and therapy.

Indications of passive immunization:

1. **To provide immediate protection**—to a nonimmune host exposed to an infection and lack active immunity to that pathogen and when there is insufficient time for active immunization to take effect.
2. Treatment of some infections.
3. **For the suppression of active immunity**—when it may be injurious, e.g., administration of anti-Rh (D) IgG to Rh-negative mother, bearing Rh-positive baby at the time of delivery to prevent isoimmunization.
4. **Immunocompromised or immunodeficient individuals,** e.g., children with hypogammaglobulinemia, individuals with AIDS, patients receiving chemotherapy, organ transplant recipients receiving immunosuppressive therapy.

Combined Immunization

Combined immunization is a combination of active and passive methods of immunization which is sometimes employed. For example, it is often undertaken in some diseases such as tetanus, diphtheria, and rabies. Passive immunity provides the protection necessary till the active immunity becomes effective.

Local Immunity

Local immunity is conferred by *secretory IgA* produced locally by plasma cells present on mucosal surfaces or in secretory glands. There appears to be a selective transport of such antibodies between the various mucosal surfaces and secretory glands.

Examples:

1. Poliomyelitis immunization
2. Influenza immunization

Herd Immunity

It is the level of resistance of a community or a group of people to a particular disease and is relevant in the control of epidemic diseases.

High level of herd immunity: Eradication of communicable diseases depends on the development of a high level of herd immunity rather than on the development of a high level of immunity in individuals.

KEY POINTS

- ❖ Innate or natural immunity—is the resistance to infections which an individual possesses by virtue of his genetic or constitutional make up.
- ❖ Acquired immunity refers to the resistance that an individual acquires during his lifetime.
- ❖ Artificial active immunity is the resistance induced by vaccines.

IMPORTANT QUESTIONS

1. Tabulate the differences between active and passive immunity.
2. Write short notes on:
    a. Innate immunity
    b. Active immunity
    c. Passive immunity

MULTIPLE CHOICE QUESTIONS (MCQs)

1. **All are acute phase proteins, *except*:**
    a. C-reactive protein
    b. Mannose binding protein
    c. Serum amyloid P component
    d. Antibody
2. **Clinical or inapparent infection leads to:**
    a. Natural active immunity
    b. Artificial active immunity
    c. Natural passive immunity
    d. Artificial passive immunity
3. **Vaccine induces:**
    a. Active natural immunity
    b. Active artificial immunity
    c. Passive natural immunity
    d. Passive artificial immunity
4. **All the following statements are true for artificial passive immunity, *except*:**
    a. Artificial passive immunity is the resistance passively transferred to a recipient by the administration of antibodies
    b. It is short lived and lasts only a few weeks to a few months
    c. This type of immunity is immediate
    d. This immunity may be induced by maternal antibodies
5. **All of the following are live vaccines, *except*:**
    a. BCG
    b. MMR
    c. Sabin vaccine
    d. TAB vaccine

Section 4: Immunology

6. All of the following are killed vaccines, *except*:
   a. Salk vaccine
   b. Non-neural vaccines for rabies
   c. Hepatitis B vaccine
   d. BCG

ANSWERS

1. d 2. a 3. b 4. d 5. d 6. d

CHAPTER 11

Immunoprophylaxis

Learning Objectives

After reading and studying this chapter, you should be able to:
- List of immunizing agents.
- Describe vaccines types and classification, storage and handling, cold chain.
- Discuss immunization schedule.
- Describe National Immunization Schedule.

■ INTRODUCTION

An important contribution of microbiology to medicine has been immunization, which is one of the most effective methods of controlling infectious diseases.

■ IMMUNIZING AGENTS

The immunizing agents may be classified as:
A. Vaccines
B. Immunoglobulins

Vaccines

A vaccine is a preparation from an infectious agent that is administered to humans and other animals to induce protective immunity against a given disease. There are two types of vaccines that induce **active** immunity: those that contain **live virus** whose pathogenicity has been **attenuated** and those that contain **killed virus**. An *attenuated* virus is one that is unable to cause disease, but retains its antigenicity and can induce protection.

Types of Vaccines

A. **Live vaccines:** Live vaccines [e.g., Bacillus Calmette-Guérin (BCG) vaccine for tuberculosis, measles, and oral polio] are prepared from live (generally attenuated) organisms. These organisms have been passed repeatedly in the laboratory in tissue culture or chick embryos and have lost their capacity to induce full blown disease but retain their immunogenicity. In general, live vaccines are more potent immunizing agents than killed vaccines.

B. **Inactivated or killed vaccines:** Organisms killed by heat or chemicals, when infected into the body stimulate active immunity. They are usually safe but generally less efficacious than live vaccines. Killed vaccines usually require a primary series of 2 or 3 doses of vaccine to produce an adequate antibody response, and in most cases "booster" injections are required. Killed vaccines are usually administered by subcutaneous or intramuscular route.

Examples of vaccines:

1. **Bacterial vaccines:** Active immunity is induced by vaccines prepared from bacteria or their products. Bacterial vaccines are composed of capsular polysaccharides, inactivated protein exotoxins (toxoids), and killed bacteria.

    There are three major types of inactivated bacterial vaccines: (1) **Toxoid** (inactivated toxins), (2) **inactivated (killed)** bacteria, and (3) surface components of the bacteria, such as **capsule or protein subunits.** Most antibacterial vaccines protect against the pathogenic action of toxins.

    Certain organisms produce exotoxins, e.g., diphtheria and tetanus bacilli. The toxins produced by these organisms are detoxicated and used in the preparation of vaccines. In general, toxoid preparations are highly efficacious and safe immunizing agents.

    Vaccines against *Haemophilus (H) influenzae* B, *Neisseria meningitidis, Salmonella typhi,* and *Streptococcus pneumonia* (23 strains) are prepared from capsular polysaccharides.

2. **Viral vaccines:** Inactivated viral vaccines: These are available for polio (injectable polio vaccine- Salk), hepatitis A, influenza, and rabies, among other viruses.

    Subunit vaccine: Consist of the **bacterial or viral components** that elicit a protective immune response, e.g., **two viral**

subunit vaccines **hepatitis B virus (HBV) vaccine** and the **human papilloma virus (HPV) vaccine** contain purified viral antigens.

C. **DNA vaccines:**
Future directions for vaccination
1. Hybrid virus vaccines
2. **Genetically engineered subunit vaccines**: Influenza, rabies, herpes simplex virus subunit vaccines
3. Peptide subunit vaccines
4. **Adjuvants** in addition to alum are being developed to enhance the immunogenicity.
5. DNA vaccines
6. **Reverse vaccinology**: A new approach, termed *reverse vaccinology*, was used to develop a vaccine for *Neisseria meningitidis* B.

The Cold Chain

The "cold chain" is a system of storage and transport of vaccines at low temperature from the manufacturer to the actual vaccination site. The cold chain system is necessary because vaccine failure may occur due to failure to store and transport under strict temperature controls. The success of national immunization program is highly dependent on supply chain system for delivery of vaccines and equipment, with a functional system that meets six rights of supply chain. The right vaccine in the right quantity at the right place at the right time in the right condition (no temperature breaks in cold chain) and at the right cost.

Cold Chain Equipment

The cold chain equipment used in Universal Immunization Program (UIP) are classified as follows:
A. Storage-electrical, solar, nonelectrical
B. Transportation

Transportation: Refrigerated vaccine van; Insulated vaccine van; and cold box vaccine carrier.

Correct Storage and Use of Diluents

Only use the diluents supplied and packaged by the manufacturer with the vaccine, since the diluent is specifically designed for the needs of that vaccine, with respect to volume, pH level and chemical properties.

Store the diluents, between +2 and +8°C in the ice-lined refrigerator (ILR). If there are constraints of space, then store diluents outside the cold chain. However, remember to cool diluents for at least 24 hours before use to ensure that vaccines and diluents are at +2° to +8°C when being reconstituted. Otherwise, it can lead to thermal shock, i.e., the death of some or all the essential live organisms in the vaccine. Store the diluents and droppers with the vaccines in the vaccine carrier during transportation. Diluents should not come in direct contact with the ice pack.

■ IMMUNIZATION

Immunization is of three types: **Active immunization, passive immunization,** and **combined passive and active immunization.**

A. Active Immunization

Active immunization is the protection of susceptible humans from communicable diseases by the administration of vaccines (vaccination).

Universal Immunization Program

In May 1974, the World Health Organization (WHO) officially launched a global immunization program, known as **Expanded Program on Immunization (EPI)** to protect all the children of the world against six vaccine—preventable diseases, namely—diphtheria, whooping cough, tetanus, polio, tuberculosis, and measles by the year 2000. EPI was launched in India in January 1978. The program is now called **Universal Child Immunization.** The Indian version, the **UIP,** was launched on November 19, 1985.

Immunization Schedules

1. **National Immunization Schedule:** The National Immunization Schedule is given in **Table 11.1.** The first visit may be made when

the infant is 6 weeks old; the second and third visits, at intervals of 1–2 months. Oral polio vaccine (OPV) may be given concurrently with OPV. BCG can be given with any of the three doses but the site for the injection should be different. The schedule also covers immunization of women during pregnancy against tetanus.
2. **WHO EPI Schedule:** The purpose is to assist health planners to develop an appropriate country specific immunization schedule based on local conditions.

TABLE 11.1: National Immunization Schedule (NIS) for infants, children, and pregnant women (India).

Vaccine	Due age	Maximum age	Dose	Diluent	Route	Site
For pregnant women						
TT-1	Early in pregnancy		0.5 mL	No	Intramuscular	Upper arm
TT-2*	4 weeks after TT-1		0.5 mL	No	Intramuscular	Upper arm
TT-booster*	If received TT doses in a pregnancy within the last 3 years		0.5 mL	No	Intramuscular	Upper arm
For infants						
Bacillus Calmette-Guerin (BCG)	At birth	Till 1 year of age	(0.05 mL until 1 month) 0.1 mL beyond age 1 month	Yes Manufacturer supplied diluent (sodium chloride)	Intradermal	Upper arm (left)
Hepatitis B Birth dose	At birth	Within 24 hours	0.5 mL	No	Intramuscular	Anterolateral side of mid-thigh (left)

Contd...

Contd...

Vaccine	Due age	Maximum age	Dose	Diluent	Route	Site
bOPV-0	At birth	Within the first 15 days	2 drops	–	Oral	Oral
bOPV-1, 2 and 3	At 6, 10, and 14 weeks	Till 5 years of age	2 drops	–	Oral	Oral
Pentavalent1, 2 and 3†‡ (Diphtheria + Pertussis + Tetanus + Hepatitis B + Hib)	At 6, 10, and 14 weeks†	1 year of age	0.5 mL	No	Intramuscular	Anterolateral side of mid-thigh (left)
Fractional inactivate poliovaccine (IPV)	At 6 and 14 weeks	1 year of age	0.1 mL	No	Intradermal	Upper arm (right)
Rotavirus‡ (where applicable)	At 6, 10 and 14 weeks	1 year of age	5 drops	No	Oral	Oral
Pneumococcal conjugate vaccine (PCV)—where applicable	At 6 and 14 weeks At 9 completed months booster	1 year of age	0.5 mL	No	Intramuscular	Anterolateral side of mid-thigh (right)
Measles/rubella 1st dose§	At 9 completed months-12 months	5 years of age	0.5 mL	Yes Manufacturer supplied diluent (sterile water)	Subcutaneous	Upper arm (right)

Contd...

Contd...

Vaccine	Due age	Maximum age	Dose	Diluent	Route	Site
Japanese encephalitis-1 (when applicable)	At 9–12 months	15 years of age	0.5 mL	Yes Manufacturer supplied diluent (phosphate buffer solution)	Subcutaneous	Upper arm (left)
Vitamin A 1st dose	At 9 months	5 years of age (1 lakh IU)	1 mL	–	Oral	Oral
For children						
DPT booster-1	16–24 months	7 years of age	0.5 mL	No	Intramuscular	Anterolateral side of mid-thigh (left)
Measles/ Rubella 2nd dose[§]	16–24 months	5 years of age	0.5 mL	Yes Manufacturer supplied diluent (sterile water)	Subcutaneous	Upper arm (right)
bOPV booster	16–24 months	5 years of age	2 drops	No	Oral	Oral
Japanese encephalitis-2[‖] (when applicable)	16–24 months*	Till 15 years of age	0.5 mL	Yes Manufacturer supplied diluent (phosphate buffer solution)	Subcutaneous	Upper arm (left)

Contd...

Contd...

Vaccine	Due age	Maximum age	Dose	Diluent	Route	Site
Vitamin A¶(2nd to 9th dose)	At 16 months. Then one dose every 6 months	Up to the age of 5 years	2 mL (2 lakh IU)	–	Oral	Oral
DPT booster-2	5–6 years	7 years of age	0.5 mL	No	Intra-muscular	Upper arm
Tetanus toxoid (TT)	10 years and 16 years	16 years	0.5 mL	No	Intra-muscular	Upper arm

*Give TT-2 or booster doses before 36 weeks of pregnancy. However, give these even if more than 36 weeks have passed. Give TT to a woman in labor, if she has not previously received TT.
† Pentavalent vaccine is introduced in place of DPT and Hep B 1, 2, and 3.
‡ Rotavirus vaccine is being introduced in phases.
§MR vaccine introduced in phases replacing measles vaccine in the UIP schedule. If first does delayed beyond 12 months ensure minimum 1 month gap between 2 MR doses.
‖ JE vaccine has been introduced in selected endemic districts. If first dose is delayed beyond 12 months ensure minimum 3 months gap between 2 JE doses.
¶The 2nd to 9th doses of vitamin A can be administered to children 1–5 years old during biannual rounds, in collaboration with ICDS.

Note:
- Human papilloma virus (HPV) vaccine—presently not in schedule.
- Tetanus diphtheria (Td) to replace TT—to be added in schedule.

B. Passive Immunization

Passive immunization is used when it is considered necessary to protect a patient at short notice and for a limited period. Antitoxic, antibacterial, or antiviral antibodies in human (homologous) or animal (heterologous) serum are injected to give temporary protection.

Preparations for passive immunization: Three types of preparations are available for passive immunization:

1. **Normal human immunoglobulin:** Normal human Ig is used to prevent measles in highly susceptible individuals and to provide temporary protection against hepatitis A infection.
2. **Specific human immunoglobulin:** These preparations are made from the plasma of patients who have recently recovered from

an infection or are obtained from individuals who have been immunized against a specific infection. They, therefore, have high antibody content against an individual infection and provide immediate protection, e.g., specific human Igs are used for passive immunization against tetanus [human tetanus immunoglobulin (HTIG)], hepatitis B (HBIG), and rabies (HRIG).
3. **Antisera:** The term *antiserum* is applied to materials prepared in animals. Originally, passive immunization was achieved by the administration of antisera or antitoxins prepared from nonhuman sources such as horses.

The current trend is in favor of using immunoglobulins wherever possible.

C. Combined Passive and Active Immunization

In some diseases (e.g., tetanus, diphtheria, and rabies) passive immunization is often undertaken in conjunction with inactivated vaccine products, to provide both immediate (but temporary) passive immunity and slowly developing active immunity. If the injections are given at separate sites, the immune response to the active agent, may or may not be impaired by immunoglobulin.

KEY POINT

Immunoprophylaxis is the prevention of disease by the production of active or passive immunity.

IMPORTANT QUESTIONS

1. Define vaccine, its type and classification.
2. Discuss cold chain and discuss the methods of safe storage and handling of vaccines.
3. Write short notes on:
    a. Live attenuated vaccines
    b. Killed vaccines
    c. Toxoids

MULTIPLE CHOICE QUESTIONS (MCQs)

1. Which of the following vaccines is/are killed vaccines?
    a. Cholera vaccine
    b. Pertussis vaccine
    c. Japanese encephalitis vaccine
    d. All of the above

2. An example of killed inactivated vaccine is:
   a. MMR vaccine
   b. Influenza vaccines
   c. Oral polio vaccine
   d. BCG vaccine
3. An example of live attenuated vaccine is:
   a. Hepatitis B vaccine
   b. Rocky Mountain spotted fever vaccine
   c. Yellow fever vaccine
   d. Rabies vaccine
4. Which of the following vaccines is/are subunit vaccine/s?
   a. Hepatitis B vaccine (plasma derived)
   b. Vi typhoid fever vaccine
   c. Meningococcal vaccine
   d. All of the above
5. Toxoid is used for active immunization against:
   a. Pertussis
   b. Diphtheria
   c. Typhoid fever
   d. Tuberculosis
6. Specific immunoglobulins are available for passive immunization against:
   a. Tetanus
   b. Rabies
   c. Hepatitis B
   d. All of the above
7. Combined passive and active immunization is available against all the diseases, *except*:
   a. Poliomyelitis
   b. Tetanus
   c. Rabies
   d. Diphtheria

ANSWERS

| 1. d | 2. b | 3. c | 4. d | 5. b | 6. d |
| 7. a | | | | | |

CHAPTER 12

Hypersensitivity Reactions

Learning Objectives

After reading and studying this chapter, you should be able to:
- Compare major types of hypersensitivity reactions.
- Differentiate between immediate and delayed hypersensitivity.
- Discuss type I, type II, type III, and type IV hypersensitivity reactions—mechanism and examples.

■ HYPERSENSITIVITY

Hypersensitivity is an exaggerated immune response that results in tissue damage and is manifested in the individual on second or subsequent contact with an antigen.

Immune responses to foreign antigens are, for the most part, beneficial to the responding individual. Nevertheless, at times the response to a seemingly innocuous antigen can result in tissue damage and even death. This inappropriate immune response is termed hypersensitivity or allergy.

■ CLASSIFICATION OF HYPERSENSITIVITY REACTIONS

Hypersensitivity reactions have been classified traditionally into "immediate" and "delayed" types, based on the time required for a sensitized host to develop clinical reactions on reexposure to the antigen.

The major differences between the immediate and delayed types of hypersensitivity reactions are shown in **Table 12.1**.

TABLE 12.1: Distinguishing features of immediate and delayed types of hypersensitivity.

Characteristic	Immediate hypersensitivity	Delayed hypersensitivity
Time of reaction after challenge with antigen	Reaction appears and recedes rapidly	Appears slowly, lasts longer
Induction	Antigens or haptens	Antigen or hapten intradermally or with by any route
Immune response	"Antibody-mediated" reaction	"Cell-mediated" reaction
Transfer of hypersensitivity	Passive transfer possible with serum	Cannot be transferred with serum; but possible with T cells or transfer factor
Desensitization	Easy, but short-lived	Difficult, but long-lasting

Gell and Coombs Classification

The Gell-Coombs classification system divides hypersensitivity into four types: I, II, III, and IV.
Type I (anaphylactic, IgE, or reagin dependent)
Type II (cytotoxic or cell stimulating)
Type III (immune complex or toxic complex disease)
Type IV (delayed or cell-mediated hypersensitivity)

The classification and some of the features of hypersensitivity reactions are shown in **Table 12.2.**

Type I Hypersensitivity (IgE Dependent)

A type I hypersensitive reaction is induced by certain types of antigens referred to as ***allergens***.

Anaphylaxis

Anaphylaxis is an inclusive term for the reactions caused when certain antigens combine with IgE antibodies. Anaphylactic responses can be:
A. **Systemic reactions:** Systemic reactions produce shock and breathing difficulties and are sometimes fatal.
B. **Localized reactions:** Localized reactions are chronic or recurrent, nonfatal, typically localized form called **atopy**.

TABLE 12.2: Comparison of major types of hypersensitivity reactions.

Type of reaction	Time required for manifestation	Mediators	Clinical syndrome
Type 1: IgE type	Minutes	IgE: Histamine and other pharmacological agents	1. Anaphylaxis 2. Atopy
Type II: Cytolytic and cytotoxic	Variable: Hours to days	IgG: IgM, complement	1. Transfusion reactions 2. Rh incompatibility
Type III: Immune complex	Variable: Hours to days	IgG: IgM, C, leukocytes	1. Arthus reaction 2. Serum sickness
Type IV: Delayed hypersensitivity	Hours to days	T cells: lymphokines; macrophages	1. Tuberculin test 2. Contact dermatitis 3. Graft rejection 4. Tumor immunity

Systemic Anaphylaxis (or Anaphylactic Shock)

Systemic anaphylaxis is a generalized response that occurs when an individual sensitized to an allergen receives a subsequent exposure to it.

Systemic anaphylaxis is a shock like and often fatal state whose onset occurs within minutes of a type I hypersensitive reaction.

Antigens: A wide range of antigens have been shown to trigger this reaction in susceptible humans, including the venom from bee, wasp, hornet, and ant stings; drugs, such as penicillin, insulin, and antitoxins; and seafood and nuts. If not treated quickly, these reactions can be fatal.

Mechanism of anaphylaxis: *The immunologic basis for hypersensitivity is cytotropic IgE antibody.*

After an initial contact with an antigen, the individual produces IgE antibodies. IgE molecules are bound to surface receptors on mast cells and basophils. These cells carry large numbers of such receptors. IgE molecules attach to these receptors by their Fc end, leaving two antigen-binding sites free. Mast cells and basophils coated by IgE are said to be sensitized, making the individual allergic to the allergen (**Fig. 12.1**).

Following exposure to the shocking dose, the antigen molecules combine with the cell bound IgE, bridging the gap between adjacent

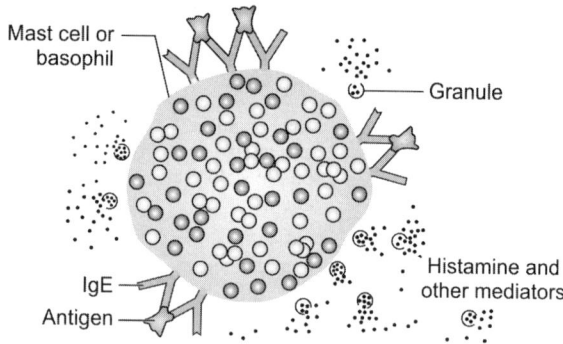

Fig. 12.1: Antigen-induced mediator release from mast cell.

antibody molecules. This cross-linking increases the permeability of the cells to calcium ions and leads to degranulation, with release of biologically active substances contained in the granules. The pharmacologically active mediators released from the granules act on the surrounding tissues. The manifestations of anaphylaxis are due to pharmacological mediators, which can be classified as two types either **primary or secondary.**

Primary mediators of anaphylaxis: The primary mediators are produced before degranulation and are stored in the granules.

1. **Histamine:** Histamine induces smooth muscle contraction in diverse tissues and organs, including vasculature, intestines, uterus, and especially the bronchioles.
2. **Heparin:** It contributes to anaphylaxis in dogs, but apparently not in human beings.
3. **Serotonin:** It induces contraction of smooth muscle, increased vascular permeability, and capillary dilatation.
4. Chemotactic factors:
    i. **Eosinophil chemotactic factor (ECF-A):** These probably contribute to the eosinophilia.
    ii. **Neutrophil chemotactic factors (NCF):** Attracts neutrophils (NCF).
5. **Proteases**: Result in increased permeability to a variety of cell types.

Secondary mediators of anaphylaxis:

1. **Platelet activating factor (PAF):** It induces a rapid wheal and flare reaction when injected into human skin.

2. **Leukotrienes and prostaglandin**—are bronchoconstrictors.
3. **Cytokines**: These cytokines leading to the recruitment of inflammatory cells.

Localized Anaphylaxis (Atopy)

The term "atopy" (literally meaning out of place or strangeness) refers to naturally occurring familial hypersensitivities of human beings. It was introduced by Coca (1923) and typified by hay fever and asthma. The antigens commonly involved in atopy are **inhalants contact allergens**, to which the skin and conjunctiva may be exposed.

Predisposition to atopy is genetically determined, genotypes. Atopy therefore runs in families.

Mechanism of Atopy

The mechanism of development of atopy is essentially the same as that of systemic anaphylaxis. The symptoms of atopy are caused by the release of pharmacologically active substances following the combination of the antigen and the cell fixed IgE.

Atopic sensitivity is due to an overproduction of IgE antibodies.

Clinical Expression of Atopic Reactions

The clinical expression of atopic reactions is usually determined by the portal of entry of the antigen-conjunctivitis, rhinitis, gastrointestinal symptoms, and dermatitis following exposure through the eyes, respiratory tract, intestine or skin, respectively.

Type II Hypersensitivity: Cytolytic and Cytotoxic

These reactions involve a combination of **IgG (or IgM) antibodies** with an antigenic determinant on the surface of cells. Antibody can activate the **complement** system, creating pores in the membrane of a foreign cell, or it can mediate cell destruction by **antibody-dependent cell-mediated cytotoxicity (ADCC)**. Type II hypersensitivity is generally called **cytolytic or cytotoxic reactions** because it results in the destruction of host cells, either by lysis or toxic mediators (**Fig. 12.2**).

Examples:
1. **Transfusion reactions:** A **transfusion reaction** can occur, if a patient receives erythrocytes differing antigenically from his or her own during blood transfusion.

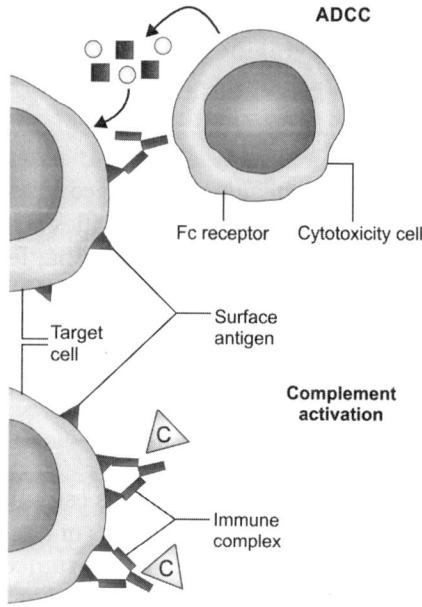

Fig. 12.2: Hypersensitivity.
(ADCC: antibody-dependent cell-mediated cytotoxicity)

2. **Hemolytic disease of the newborn:** If the child is Rh+ and mother Rh− will cross the placenta and destroy fetal RBCs.
3. **Drug-induced cytotoxic reactions:** Blood platelets (thrombocytes) that are destroyed by drug-induced cytotoxic reactions in the disease called **thrombocytopenic purpura** (quinine is a familiar example). Immune caused destruction of granulocytic white cells is called **agranulocytosis.** When RBCs are destroyed in the same manner, the condition is termed **hemolytic anemia.**
4. Anemia due to infectious diseases.

Type III Hypersensitivity: Immune Complex-mediated

Type III reactions involve antibodies against soluble antigens circulating in the serum. The antigen-antibody complexes are deposited in organs and cause inflammatory damage. The tissue damage that results from the deposition of immune complexes is caused by the activation of complement, platelets, and phagocytes; in essence, an acute inflammatory response.

Models of Immune Complex-mediated Disease

Two basic models of immune complex-mediated disease have been well-characterized: **The Arthus reaction** and **serum sickness**.

Arthus Reaction (Local Immune Complex Disease)

A localized form of experimental immune complex-mediated vasculitis is called **Arthus reaction**. This is a local manifestation of generalized hypersensitivity.

Serum Sickness (Systemic Immune Complex Disease)

This is a systemic form of type III hypersensitivity. When large amounts of antigen enter the bloodstream and bind to antibody, circulating immune complexes can form. If antigen is in excess, small complexes form, they can cause tissue damaging type III reactions at various sites. This appears 7-12 days following a single injection of a high concentration of foreign serum such as the diphtheria antitoxin.

Pathogenesis: The pathogenesis is the formation of immune complexes (consisting of the foreign serum and antibody to it that reaches high enough titers by 7-12 days) and the circulating immune complexes deposit in the blood vessel walls and tissues, leading to increased vascular permeability and thus to inflammatory diseases such as glomerulonephritis and arthritis. Antigen-antibody aggregates can fix **complement** leading to **inflammation** and **tissue damage**.

Diseases Associated with Immune Complexes

- Systemic lupus erythematosus
- Rheumatoid arthritis
- Poststreptococcal glomerulonephritis
- Dengue hemorrhagic fever

Type IV Hypersensitivity: Delayed Hypersensitivity

Type IV hypersensitivity reactions (delayed hypersensitivity) constitute one aspect of cell-mediated immune response and are caused mainly by T cells. These are typically provoked by intracellular microbial infections or haptens and consist of a mixed cellular reaction involving lymphocytes and macrophages in particular. It is named delayed hypersensitivity because it appears in 24-48 hours

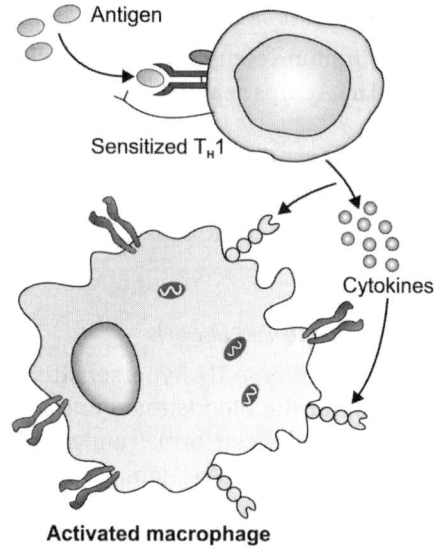

Fig. 12.3: Type IV (delayed or cell-mediated hypersensitivity).

after the presensitized host encounters the antigen, while immediate hypersensitivity reactions develop in 0.5–12 hours (**Fig. 12.3**).

Delayed hypersensitivity cannot be passively transferred by serum but can be transferred by lymphocytes or the transfer factor.

Types of Delayed Hypersensitivity

Two types of delayed hypersensitivity are recognized: The tuberculin (infection) type and the contact dermatitis type.

1. **Tuberculin (infection) type:** In tuberculin hypersensitivity, tuberculin or purified protein derivative (PPD) is injected into the skin of the forearm. Intradermally, in an individual sensitized to tuberculoprotein by prior infection or immunization. An indurated (firm and hard) inflammatory reaction, 10 mm or more in diameter, develops at the site of injection within 48–72 hours. It is characterized by erythema due to increased blood flow to the damaged area and the infiltration with a large number of mononuclear cells, mainly T lymphocytes and about 10–20% macrophages into the injection site are responsible for the induration.

The tuberculin test; therefore, provides useful indication of the state of delayed hypersensitivity (cell-mediated immunity) to the bacilli. Tuberculin type hypersensitivity develops in many infections with bacteria, fungi, viruses, and parasites.

2. **Contact dermatitis type:** Allergic contact dermatitis is caused by haptens that combine with proteins in the skin to form the allergen that elicits the immune response.

   Examples: Examples of these haptens include cosmetics, plant materials topical chemotherapeutic agents, metals (nickel and chromium), and chemicals.

Type V Hypersensitivity (Stimulatory Type): Jones-Mote Reaction (or) Cutaneous Basophil Hypersensitivity

This is an antibody-mediated hypersensitivity and is a modification of Type II hypersensitivity reaction.

Shwartzman Reaction

This is not an immune reaction but rather a perturbation in factors affecting intravascular coagulation.

KEY POINT

Hypersensitivity is an exaggerated immune response that results in tissue damage and is manifested in the individual on second or subsequent contact with an antigen. Hypersensitivity reactions are of five types: Types I, II, III, IV, and V.

IMPORTANT QUESTIONS

1. What is hypersensitivity? How do you classify various types of hypersensitivity reactions? Describe type I hypersensitivity reactions.
2. Write short notes on:
   a. Anaphylaxis
   b. Atopy
   c. Type III hypersensitivity (or) immune complex diseases
   d. Arthus reaction
   e. Serum sickness
   f. Type IV hypersensitivity (or) delayed-type hypersensitivity (DTH)

MULTIPLE CHOICE QUESTIONS (MCQs)

1. All the following statements are true for type I hypersensitivity reaction, *except*:
   a. It is called immediate hypersensitivity reaction
   b. It always involves IgE-mediated degranulation of basophils or mast cells
   c. This reaction is always rapid
   d. Atopy is one of the manifestation
2. All are primary mediators of anaphylaxis, *except*:
   a. Histamine
   b. Proteases
   c. Eosinophil chemotactic factors of anaphylaxis
   d. Platelet activating factor
3. Schultz-Dale phenomenon is an example of:
   a. Type I hypersensitivity reaction
   b. Type II hypersensitivity reaction
   c. Type III hypersensitivity reaction
   d. Type IV hypersensitivity reaction
4. All the followings diseases are true for Arthus reaction, *except*:
   a. It is a local manifestation of generalized hyper-sensitivity
   b. The tissue damage is due to formation of local precipitating immune complexes
   c. This is systemic form of type II hypersensitivity
   d. It manifests after a single injection of a high concentration of foreign serum
5. All of the following diseases are true for serum sickness, *except*:
   a. It manifests after a single injection of a high concentration of foreign serum
   b. Disease is self-limited
   c. This is systemic form of type II hypersensitivity
   d. It is a localized inflammatory reaction due to deposition of immune complexes
6. Delayed hypersensitivity reaction is mediated by:
   a. T lymphocytes
   b. B lymphocytes
   c. Macrophages
   d. Basophils

7. Shwartzman reaction is an example of:
   a. Type I hypersensitivity reaction
   b. Type II hypersensitivity reaction
   c. Type III hypersensitivity reaction
   d. None of the above

ANSWERS
1. b   2. d   3. c   4. d   5. d   6. a
7. d

CHAPTER 13

Autoimmunity

Learning Objectives

After reading and studying this chapter, you should be able to:
- Describe the mechanisms of autoimmunity.
- Classify autoimmune diseases.
- List autoimmune diseases.

■ INTRODUCTION

One of the classically accepted features of the immune system is the capacity to distinguish self from nonself. Normally, a person is tolerized to self-antigens during the development of the immune system as a fetus and later in life by other mechanisms (e.g., oral tolerization).

■ DEFINITION

Autoimmunity is a condition in which structural or functional damage is produced by the action of immunologically competent cells or antibodies against the normal components of the body. Autoimmunity is due to copious production of autoantibodies and autoreactive T cells.

■ MECHANISMS OF AUTOIMMUNITY

A variety of mechanisms have been proposed for induction of autoimmunity.
1. **Forbidden clones:** During embryonic life, clones of cells that have immunological reactivity with self-antigens are eliminated. Such clones are called **forbidden clones**. Their persistence

or development in later life by somatic mutation can lead to autoimmunity.
2. **Neoantigens or altered antigens:** Cells or tissues may undergo antigenic alteration as a result of physical, chemical or biological influences. Such altered or "neoantigens" may elicit an immune response.
3. **Molecular mimicry:** The fortuitous similarity between some foreign and self-antigens is the basis of the "cross reacting antigens" theory of autoimmunity.
4. Polyclonal B-cell activation
5. Activity of helper and suppressor T-cells
6. **Sequestered antigens:** Certain self-antigens are present in closed systems and are not accessible to the immune apparatus. These are known as **sequestered antigens**, e.g., **(i) Lens antigen of the eye; (ii) Sperm antigens; (iii) Heart muscle antigens.**
7. Defects in the idiotype-anti-idiotype network
8. Genetic factors

■ CLASSIFICATION OF AUTOIMMUNE DISEASES

Based on the site of involvement and nature of lesions, autoimmune diseases may be classified as:
A. Localized (or organ specific), e.g., Hashimoto's thyroiditis (self-antigen is thyroid proteins and cell; immune response autoantibodies).
B. Systemic (or nonorgan specific), e.g., rheumatoid arthritis (self-antigen is connective tissue, IgG; immune response is autoantibodies, immune complexes).

KEY POINT

Autoimmunity is a condition in which structural or functional damage is produced by the action of immunologically competent cells or antibodies against the normal components of the body.

IMPORTANT QUESTIONS

1. What is autoimmunity? What are the mechanisms of autoimmune diseases giving suitable examples?

2. Write briefly on:
   a. Autoimmunity
   b. Mechanisms of autoimmune diseases

MULTIPLE CHOICE QUESTIONS (MCQs)

1. Lens protein of eye is an example of:
   a. Sequestered antigen
   b. Neoantigen
   c. Cross reacting antigen
   d. Molecular mimicry
2. All of the following diseases are examples of organ-specific autoimmune diseases, *except*:
   a. Goodpasture's syndrome
   b. Graves' disease
   c. Insulin-dependent diabetes mellitus
   d. Systemic lupus erythematosus

ANSWERS

1. a   2. d

CHAPTER 14

Principles and Uses of Serological Tests

Learning Objectives

After reading and studying this chapter, you should be able to:
- Describe various types of precipitation reactions and their uses.
- Discuss principle and applications of agglutination reactions.
- Describe principle and types of immunodiffusion.
- Describe principle and uses of complement fixation test.
- Discuss principle and clinical applications of immunofluorescence technique.
- Discuss principle, various types and clinical applications of ELISA techniques.

■ SEROLOGIC DIAGNOSIS

Immunologic techniques are used to detect, identify, and quantitate antigen in clinical samples, as well as to evaluate the antibody response to infection and a person's history of exposure to infectious agents. The specificity of the antibody-antigen interaction and the sensitivity of many of the immunologic techniques make them powerful laboratory tools.

Serological Tests

The study of antigen-antibody reactions in vitro is called *serology* (serum and–ology). Antigen-antibody reactions in vitro are known as serological reactions. Various types of antigen-antibody reactions are shown in **Box 14.1**.

A. Precipitation Reactions

Principle: When a soluble antigen combines with its antibody in the presence of electrolytes (NaCl) at a suitable temperature and pH, the antigen-antibody complex forms an insoluble **precipitate** and is called **precipitation**. Antibodies that thus aggregate soluble antigens are called **precipitins**.

> **Box 14.1:** Types of antigen and antibody reactions.
>
> A. Precipitation reactions
> B. Agglutination reactions
> C. Complement fixation test (CFT)
> D. Neutralization tests
> E. Opsonization
> F. Immunofluorescence
> G. Radioimmunoassay (RIA)
> H. Enzyme-linked immunosorbent assay (ELISA)
> I. Enzyme-linked fluorescent immunoassay (ELFA)
> J. Chemiluminescence-linked immunoassay (CLIA)
> K. Immunoblotting techniques
> L. Rapid tests
> – Lateral flow assay (Immunochromatographic test)
> – Flow through assay
> M. Immunoelectronmicroscopic tests

Flocculation: When instead of sedimenting, the precipitate remains suspended as floccules, the reaction is known as **flocculation**. Precipitation can take place in liquid media or in gels such as agar, agarose, or polyacrylamide.

Uses of precipitation and flocculation tests (Table 14.1).

A. **Ring test:**
   i. Ascoli's thermoprecipitin test
   ii. The grouping of streptococci by the Lancefield technique.
B. **Slide test (slide flocculation test):** Venereal Disease Research Laboratory (VDRL) test for syphilis.
C. **Tube test (tube flocculation test):** The Kahn test for syphilis.
D. **Immunodiffusion (precipitation reactions in gels)**
   Principle: Immunodiffusion refers to a precipitation reaction that occurs between an antibody and antigen in an agar gel medium. Immunodiffusion is usually performed in a soft (1%) agar gel.
   Types of immunodiffusion tests:
   1 Single diffusion in two dimensions (radial immunodiffusion—Mancini method)—can be used to detect and quantify an antigen.
   2 **Ouchterlony immuno-double-diffusion** technique is used for Elek test for toxigenicity in diphtheria bacilli.
   3 **Immunoelectrophoresis:**
      Uses:
         i. To separate many antigens
         ii. To separate the major blood proteins in serum for certain diagnostic tests—this assay is used
         iii. For testing for normal and abnormal proteins in serum and urine

TABLE 14.1: Various precipitation reactions and their uses.

Tests	Uses
A. Ring test	❖ Ascoli's thermoprecipitin test ❖ The grouping of streptococci by the Lancefield technique
B. Slide test (slide flocculation test)	Venereal Disease Research Laboratory (VDRL) test for syphilis
C. Tube test (tube flocculation test)	The Kahn test for syphilis
D. Immunodiffusion (precipitation reactions in gels)	
1. Single diffusion in two dimensions (radial immunodiffusion—Mancini method)	To detect and quantify an antigen
2. Ouchterlony immuno–double-diffusion technique	For Elek test for toxigenicity in diphtheria bacilli
3. Immunoelectrophoresis	i. To separate many antigens ii. To separate the major blood proteins in serum for certain diagnostic tests—this assay is used iii. For testing for normal and abnormal proteins in serum and urine
4. Counterimmunoelectrophoresis (CIE)	i. For detection hepatitis B surface antigen (HBs antigen) and alpha-fetoprotein in serum and meningococcal and cryptococcal antigens in CSF ii. To detect anti-DNA antibody in with several autoimmune disorders
5. Rocket electrophoresis	Quantitative estimation of antigens

4. **Counterimmunoelectrophoresis (CIE):**
   Uses:
   i. For detection of hepatitis B surface antigen (HBs antigen) and alpha-fetoprotein in serum and meningococcal and cryptococcal antigens in CSF.
   ii. To detect anti-DNA antibody in with several autoimmune disorders.
5. **Rocket electrophoresis:**
   Use: Quantitative estimation of antigens

B. Agglutination Reactions

Principle: When a particulate antigen is mixed with its antibody in the presence of electrolytes at a suitable temperature and pH, the particles are **clumped or agglutinated**. When antigen is present on the surface of a cell or particle, the addition of antibody causes a **clumping or agglutination** of the cells. Antibodies that produce such reactions are called **agglutinin**.

Applications of Agglutination Reaction (Table 14.2)
1. **Slide agglutination**
2. **Tube agglutination:**
   Uses of tube agglutination: Tube agglutination is routinely employed for the serological diagnosis of typhoid, brucellosis, and typhus fever **(Table 14.2)**.
3. **Antiglobulin (Coombs') test**
   Principle of the antiglobulin test: When sera containing incomplete anti-Rh antibodies are mixed with Rh positive red

TABLE 14.2: Various agglutination reactions and their uses.

Tests	Uses
1. Slide agglutination	❖ For the identification of unknown bacterial cultures, such as *Salmonella* and *Shigella* ❖ **Very rapid:** It is very rapid and requires only small quantities of culture and serum ❖ Also the method for blood grouping and cross matching
2. Tube agglutination	❖ **Widal test:** Widal test is used for the diagnosis of enteric fever, two types of antigens are used: the flagellar antigens (H) and somatic (O) antigen. ❖ **Tube agglutination test for brucellosis** ❖ **Weil-Felix reaction**—for serodiagnosis of **typhus fevers** is heterophil agglutination test ❖ **Paul-Bunnell test:** Infectious mononucleosis
3. Antiglobulin (Coombs') test	For demonstrating any type of incomplete or nonagglutinating antibody, as, e.g., in brucellosis

4. Passive (indirect) agglutination test	❖ **Hemagglutination test**
	  – **Rose-Waaler test**—for rheumatoid arthritis
	  – *Treponema pallidum* **hemagglutination (TPHA)**—for serological diagnosis of treponemal infection
	❖ **Latex agglutination test** (latex fixation tests)—for the detection of antistreptolysin-O (ASO), C reactive protein (CRP), RA factor, human chorionic gonadotropin (hCG) and many other antigens
	❖ **Coagglutination:**
	  – For detecting antigens in serum, urine, and CSF
	  – Identification of antigens of various streptococcal groups, *Streptococcus pneumoniae*; *Neisseria meningitidis*; *N. gonorrheae*; and *Haemophilus influenzae* types A to F grown in culture

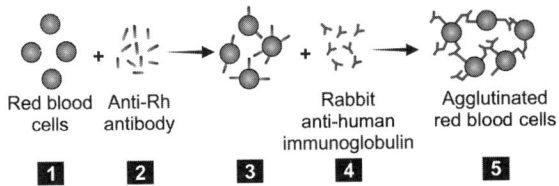

Fig. 14.1: Antiglobulin (Coombs') test. Rh positive erythrocytes; (1) are mixed with incomplete antibody; (2) The antibody coats the cells; (3) but, being incomplete, cannot produce agglutination. On addition of antiglobulin serum; (4) which is complete antibody to immunoglobulin, agglutination takes place (5).

cells, the antibody coats the surface of the erythrocytes but they are not agglutinated, when such antibody-coated erythrocytes are washed to free all unattached protein and are treated with a rabbit antihuman antiserum against human gammaglobulin (antiglobulin or Coombs' serum) the cells are agglutinated. This is the principle of the antiglobulin test **(Fig. 14.1)**.

4. **Passive (indirect) agglutination test**
   Principle: A precipitation reaction can be converted into agglutination reaction by coating soluble antigen on to the surface of **carrier particles.**
   Reversed passive agglutination: When instead of antigen, the antibody is adsorbed to carrier particles in tests for estimation of antigens, the technique is known as **reversed passive agglutination.**
   Example of passive (indirect) agglutination test:
   1. Hemagglutination test
   2. Latex agglutination test
   3. Coagglutination
   Principle: Similar to latex agglutination, coagglutination uses antibody bound to a particle to enhance visibility of the agglutination reaction between antigen and antibody Protein A on the *Staphylococcus aureus* cell wall binds the Fc portion of the immunoglobulin molecule, leaving the Fab portion free to bind antigen. Visible agglutination of the staphylococcal cells serves as a positive test to indicate antigen-antibody binding.

C. Complement Fixation Test (CFT)

Principle: When complement binds to an antigen-antibody complex, it becomes "fixed" and "used up".

Positive CF test shows absence of lysis and negative CF test shows lysis of the indicator cells.

Uses:
1. Diagnosis of syphilis
2. Diagnosis of certain viral, fungal, rickettsial, chlamydial, and protozoan diseases

D. Neutralization Tests

A. Viral Neutralization

Principle: Neutralization of viruses by their antibodies can be demonstrated in various systems. IgG, IgM, and IgA antibodies can bind to some viruses during their extracellular phase and inactivate them. This antibody-mediated viral inactivation is called **viral neutralization**.

B. Toxin Neutralization

Principle: Bacterial exotoxins are good antigens and their activity may be completely neutralized by appropriate concentrations of specific antibody.

Uses:
1. **Toxigenicity test:** To assay neutralizing capacity of an antitoxin.
2. **Schick test:** With the diphtheria toxin.
3. **Toxin neutralization in vitro**
    i. **Antistreptolysin-O (ASO) test** of the patient suffering from *Streptococcus pyogenes* infection
    ii. **Nagler's reaction:** For *Clostridium perfringens*
    iii. **Agar gel precipitation test:** To detect production of toxin by *Corynebacterium diphtheriae.*

E. Opsonization

Principle: Opsonization is the process in which microorganisms or other particles are coated by antibody and/or complement, and thus prepared for "recognition" and ingestion by phagocytic cells.

Uses: Soluble immune complexes, viruses, and tumor cells are removed.

F. Immunofluorescence

Principle: Immunofluorescence is a process in which dyes called fluorochromes are exposed to UV, violet, or blue light to make them fluoresce or emit visible light. Fluorescent dyes can be conjugated to antibodies and that such "labeled" antibodies can be used and identify antigens in tissues.

Uses:
1. **Direct immunofluorescence:** To diagnose rabies virus
2. **Indirect immunofluorescence:** Uses for diagnosis of syphilis

G. Radioimmunoassay

Principle: The principle of radioimmunoassay (RIA) is based on competitive binding of radiolabeled antigen (e.g., ^{125}I) and unlabeled antigen to a high-affinity antibody. The labeled and unlabeled (test) antigens compete for the limited binding sites on the antibody. This competition is determined by the level of the unlabeled (test) antigen present in reacting system.

Uses: For measuring hormones, serum proteins, drugs, and vitamins.

H. Enzyme-linked Immunosorbent Assay (ELISA)

Enzyme-linked immunosorbent assay, commonly known as ELISA or EIA), uses an enzyme which is linked to an antibody and used to detect and measure other antibodies or antigens. An enzyme conjugated with antibody reacts with a colourless substrate to generate a colored reaction product and the conversion of the substrate from colorless to color is a measure of antigen-antibody interaction.

Principle: Solid phase immunoassay refers to the binding of either **antigen or antibody** to a variety of solid materials.

Types of ELISA (Figs. 14.2A to C)
1. Indirect ELISA
2. Sandwich ELISA
3. Competitive ELISA
4. IgM antibody capture (MAC) ELISA
5. ELISPOT test: A modification of the ELISA assay.

I. Enzyme-linked fluorescent immunoassay (ELFA)
J. Chemiluminescence-linked immunoassay (CLIA)

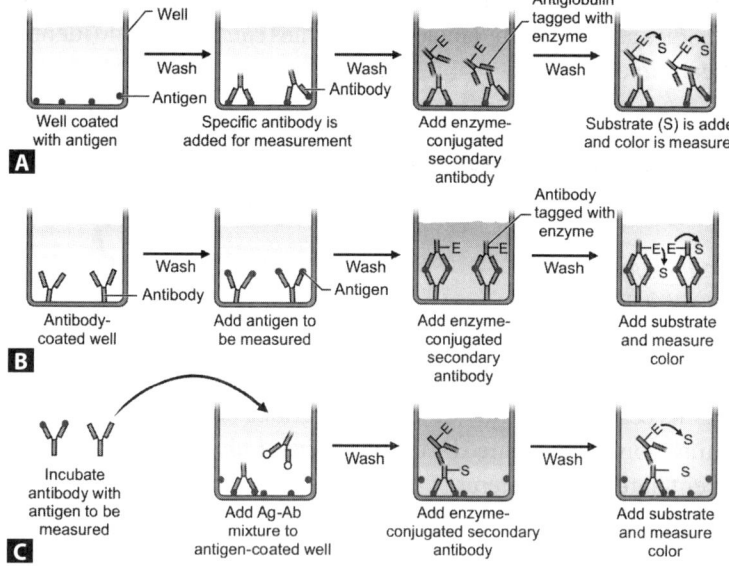

Figs. 14.2A to C: Types of enzyme-linked immunosorbent assay: (A) Indirect ELISA; (B) Sandwich ELISA; (C) Competitive ELISA (ELISA).

Uses of ELISA (Table 14.3)

TABLE 14.3: Uses of ELISA.

Parasite	Bacteria	Viruses
Entameba histolytica antigens in feces. Toxoplasma antigens in the patient serum.	Haemophilus influenzae antigens in spinal fluid. ❖ β-hemolytic streptococcal antigen in spinal fluid. ❖ Labile enterotoxin of Escheria coli in stools. To detect antibody specific for: Mycoplasmas, Chlamydiae, Borrelia burgdorferi	**To detect antibody specific for:** ❖ Hepatitis virus antigens ❖ Herpes simplex viruses 1 and 2 ❖ Respiratory syncytial virus (RSV), Cytomegalovirus, Human immunodeficiency virus (HIV), Rubella virus (both IgG and IgM), Adenovirus antigens in nasopharyngeal specimens

K. Immunoblotting Techniques

Western Blot

Principle: In this technique, viral proteins separated by electrophoresis according to their molecular weight or charge are transferred (blotted) onto a filter paper (e.g., nitrocellulose, nylon). When exposed to a patient's serum, the immobilized proteins capture virus-specific antibody and are visualized with an enzyme-conjugated antihuman antibody. This technique shows the proteins recognized by the patient serum. The position of the band on the paper indicates the antigen with which the antibody has reacted.

Uses: Western blot analysis is used to confirm ELISA results in patients suspected to be infected with the HIV.

L. Rapid Tests

1. Lateral flow assay (immunochromatographic test)
   Application: For HBsAg test, HCV Ab test, HIV Ab test, and Urine pregnancy test.
2. Flow through assay, e.g., HIV TRIDOT detects antibodies to HIV-1 and 2 separately in patient's serum.

M. Immunoelectronmicroscopic Tests

1. **Immunoelectronmicroscopy**
   Principle: When viral particles mixed with specific antisera are observed under the electron microscope, they are seen to be clumped. This is known as immune electron microscopy.
   Uses: In the study of hepatitis A virus and the viruses causing diarrhea.
2. **Immunoferritin test**
   Principle: Ferritin (an electron-dense substance from horse spleen) can be conjugated with antibody, and such labeled antibody reacting with an antigen can be visualized under the electron microscope.
3. **Immunoenzyme test**
   Principle: Some stable enzymes, such as peroxidase, can be conjugated with antibodies. Tissue sections carrying the corresponding antigens are treated with peroxidase labeled antisera. If the tissue section possesses specific antigen then

peroxidase bound to the antigen can be visualized under the electron microscope, by microhistochemical methods.
Use: Tissue sections.

KEY POINTS

- Precipitation test is a type of antigen-antibody reaction, in which the antigen occurs in a soluble form. Immunodiffusion procedures are precipitation reactions carried out in an agar gel medium. Electrophoresis can be combined with precipitation in gels in a technique called **immunoelectrophoresis.** Immunoelectrophoresis combines electrophoresis with immunodiffusion for the analysis of serum proteins.
- **Agglutination reactions:** The interaction of particulate antigens with antibodies leads to agglutination reactions. Direct agglutination reactions can be: slide agglutination test, tube agglutination test, heterophile agglutination tests and antiglobulin (Coombs') test. Passive agglutination reaction depending on the carrier particles used.
- **Complement-fixation reactions** are serological tests based on the depletion of a fixed amount of complement in the presence of an antigen-antibody reaction and: are (i) complement fixation test; (ii) immune adherence test; (iii) immobilization test; (iv) cytolytic or cytocidal reactions.
- **Neutralization reactions:** In neutralization reactions, the harmful effects of a bacterial exotoxin or virus are eliminated by a specific antibody.
- Opsonization is immune opsonization or nonimmune opsonization.
- **Immunofluorescence:** Direct immunofluorescence test is used to detect unknown antigen in a cell or tissue. Indirect immunofluorescence test is used for detection of specific antibodies in the serum and other body fluids.
- RIA is a highly sensitive and quantitative procedure that utilizes radioactively labeled antigen or antibody.
- The ELISA depends on an enzyme-substrate reaction that generates a colored reaction product.
- Western blotting is done for the detection of proteins.

Chapter 14: Principles and Uses of Serological Tests

IMPORTANT QUESTIONS

1. Name various antigen-antibody reactions. Describe the principle and applications of precipitation reactions giving suitable examples.
2. Define agglutination reaction. Discuss the principle and applications of agglutination reactions giving suitable examples.
3. Write short notes on:
   a. Immunodiffusion (or) gel diffusion
   b. Immunoelectrophoresis
   c. Counterimmunoelectrophoresis (CIEP) or counter current electrophoresis
   d. Rocket electrophoresis
   e. Coagglutination
   f. Neutralization tests
   g. Opsonization
   h. Immunofluorescence tests
   i. Radioimmunoassay (RIA)
   j. ELISA—its principle and application

MULTIPLE CHOICE QUESTIONS (MCQs)

1. The prozone phenomenon is:
   a. Zone of antibody excess
   b. Zone of antigen excess
   c. Zone of equivalence of antigens and antibody
   d. None of the above
2. Which immunoglobulin class is the most efficient to produce agglutination reaction?
   a. IgG b. IgM
   c. IgA d. IgE
3. Which immunoglobulin class is the most efficient to produce precipitation reaction?
   a. IgG b. IgM
   c. IgD d. IgE
4. Ring test is used for:
   a. C-reactive protein test
   b. Streptococcal grouping of Lancefield technique
   c. Both of the above
   d. None of the above
5. VDRL test is an example of:
   a. Agglutination test b. Flocculation test
   c. Immunofluorescence d. All of the above

6. Radial immunodiffusion can be used to estimate the following immunoglobulin classes:
   a. IgG
   b. IgM
   c. IgA
   d. All of the above
7. Counterimmunoelectrophoresis is used for detecting:
   a. Hepatitis B antigens
   b. Cryptococcal antigens
   c. *Neisseria meningitidis*
   d. All of the above
8. Tube agglutination test is used for serological diagnosis of:
   a. Enteric fever
   b. Infectious mononucleosis
   c. Typhus fever
   d. All of the above
9. Which of the following is/are example/s of heterophile agglutination test?
   a. Weil–Felix reaction
   b. Paul–Bunnell test
   c. *Streptococcus* MG agglutination test
   d. All of the above
10. Which of the following is/are example/s of passive agglutination test?
    a. Latex agglutination test
    b. Hemagglutination test
    c. Coagglutination
    d. All of the above
11. Which of the following is/are example/s of neutralization test?
    a. Schick test
    b. Antistreptolysin "O" test
    c. Nagler reaction
    d. All of the above
12. Direct immunofluorescence test may be used for detection of:
    a. Rabies virus antigens
    b. Antibodies in syphilis
    c. Both of the above
    d. None of the above
13. Indirect immunofluorescence test may be used for detection of:
    a. Rabies virus antigens
    b. Antibodies in syphilis
    c. Both of the above
    d. None of the above
14. ELISA can be used for detection of antigens and for antibodies in:
    a. HIV
    b. Rotavirus
    c. Hepatitis B virus
    d. All of the above
15. The technique of immunoblotting to analyze RNA is named as:
    a. Southern blot
    b. Northern blot
    c. Western blot
    d. None of the above

ANSWERS

1. a	2. b	3. a	4. c	5. b	6. d	
7. d	8. d	9. d	10. d	11. d	12. a	
13. b	14. d	15. b				

SECTION 5: The Control and Destruction of Microorganisms

Section Outline

- ❖ Sterilization and Disinfection
- ❖ Antimicrobial Chemotherapy
- ❖ Biomedical Waste Management

CHAPTER 15

Sterilization and Disinfection

Learning Objectives

After reading and studying this chapter, you should be able to:
- Classify and describe the different methods of sterilization and disinfection.
- Discuss the application of the different methods in the laboratory, in clinical and surgical practice.
- Choose the most appropriate method of sterilization and disinfection to be used in specific situations in the laboratory, in clinical and surgical practice.
- Describe the following: Aseptic techniques, Spaulding's classification, environment cleaning, equipment cleaning.

■ INTRODUCTION

Sterilization: Sterilization is defined as the process by which an article, surface, or medium is freed of all living microorganisms either in the vegetative or spore state.

Disinfection: Disinfection is the killing, inhibition, or removal of microorganisms that may cause disease.

Antiseptics: **Antiseptics** are chemical agents applied to tissue to prevent infection by killing or inhibiting pathogen growth; they also reduce the total microbial population.

Cleaning: The removal of visible soil (e.g., organic and inorganic material) from objects and surfaces and normally is accomplished manually or mechanically using water with detergents or enzymatic products.

■ METHODS OF STERILIZATION AND DISINFECTION (BOX 15.1)

A. Physical agents
B. Chemical agents

> **Box 15.1:** Methods of sterilization and disinfection.
>
> A. **Physical agents**
>   1. **Heat**
>   a. **Dry heat:**
>   i. Incineration—at temperature of 870–980°C
>   ii. Red heat
>   iii. Flaming
>   iv. Hot air sterilizer
>   b. **Moist heat:**
>   i. At temperature below 100°C: Pasteurization, vaccine production, inspissation, water bath
>   ii. At a temperature of 100°C: Boiling steaming, Tyndallisation
>   iii. At temperature above 100°C: Autoclave
>   2. **Filtration:** 0.22–0.45 μm pore size; high efficiency particle air (HEPA)
>   3. **Radiation:**
>   i. **Nonionizing:** Infrared and ultraviolet rays are of nonionizing type
>   ii. **Ionizing radiation:** These include X-rays, γ (gamma) rays, and cosmic rays
>   4. **Ultrasonic and sonic vibrations:** Variable exposure to 254-nm wavelength
> B. **Chemical agents**
>   1. **Surface-active disinfectants:** Quaternary ammonium compounds (quats) and soap
>   2. **Phenol and phenolics:** Cresol, chlorhexidine, chloroxylenol, and hexachlorophene
>   3. **Halogens:** Iodine, chlorine
>   4. **Alcohols:** Ethyl alcohol (ethanol) and isopropyl alcohol
>   5. **Heavy metal derivatives:** Mercury, silver, arsenic, zinc, and copper
>   6. **Chemical food preservatives:** Organic acids nitrate/nitrites
>   7. **Aldehydes:** Formaldehyde, glutaraldehyde, ortho-phthalaldehyde
>   8. **Chemical sterilization:**
>   ◊ Ethylene oxide and other gaseous sterilants
>   ◊ Plasma sterilization
>   ◊ Supercritical fluids
>   9. **Peroxygens and other forms of oxygen** peroxygens, hydrogen peroxide, peracetic acid (peroxyacetic acid, or PAA), ozone (O_3)

A. Physical Agents

1. Heat

Heat is the most reliable and universally applicable method of sterilization. Either **dry or moist heat** may be applied.

Mechanism of action

a. *Dry heat:* The lethal effect of dry heat or desiccation in general, is usually due to **protein denaturation, oxidative damage,** and

toxic effects of elevated levels of **electrolytes**.
b. *Moist heat:* Kills microorganisms by **coagulation and denaturation of their enzymes** and **structural proteins**.

a. Dry Heat Sterilization

i. **Incineration:** By this method, infective material is reduced to ashes, such as pathological waste materials, surgical dressings, contaminated material, animal carcasses, and other clinical waste are safely destroyed by incineration.

ii. **Red heat:** Inoculating wires loops and points of forceps are sterilized by holding them almost vertically in a Bunsen flame until red hot.

iii. **Flaming:** Scalpel blades, glass slides, mouth of culture tubes, and bottles are exposed to a flame for a few seconds.

iv. **Hot air sterilizer:** Hot air sterilizer is the most widely used method of sterilization by dry heat. It is used to process materials, which can withstand high temperatures for length of time needed for sterilization by dry heat, but which are likely to be affected by contact with steam. Hot air oven is electrically heated, with heating. It should be fitted with a fan to provide forced air circulation throughout the oven chamber, a temperature indicator, a control thermostat and timer, open-mesh shelving, and adequate wall insulation.

Preparation of load

1. **No overloading:** It must **not be overloaded** and the individual articles or packs of the load are positioned to allow free circulation of hot air between and around the item.
2. **Articles**: Should be thoroughly **clean and dry.**
3. **Glassware:** Should be perfectly **dry before being placed in the oven.**
4. **Test tubes and flasks**: Should be **wrapped in paper.**
5. **Rubber materials**, except silicon rubber, will not withstand the sterilizing temperature.
6. **Cotton plugs:** May get charred at 180°C.
7. **Heat-sensitive materials:** Dry heat sterilization is slow and not suitable for heat-sensitive materials like many plastic and rubber items.

Sterilizing cycle

The sterilization hold time—is set to **160°C for 2 hours or 170°C for 1 hour, or 180°C for 30 minutes.**

Uses of hot air oven
It is a method of choice for sterilization of:
1. **Glassware**—such as tubes, flasks, measuring cylinders, all-glass syringes, glass petri dishes, and glass pipettes.
2. **Metal instruments**—such as forceps, scissors, and scalpels.
3. **Nonaqueous materials and powders, oils and greases** in sealed containers and swab sticks packed in test tubes.

Sterilization Controls
A. **Biological control:** An envelope containing a filter paper strip impregnated with spores of *Bacillus subtilis* subsp. *niger* is inserted into suitable packs. No growth of *Bacillus subtilis* subsp *niger* indicates proper sterilization.
B. **Chemical indicator:** A chemical indicator, such as **Browne's tubes No. 3** containing red solution is inserted in each load and a color change from red to green is observed, which indicates proper sterilization.
C. **Thermocouples**: Thermocouples may also be used periodically.

b. Moist Heat (Box 15.1)

i. At a Temperature Below 100°C

Pasteurization of milk: Disinfection by moist heat at temperature below 100°C is termed as **pasteurization.** Milk can be pasteurized in two ways. The temperature is employed either **63°C for 30 minutes** (holder **method**) or **72°C for 15–20 seconds** (the **flash method**) followed by **rapid cooling to 13°C or lower.**
a. Vaccine preparation
b. **Inspissation:** Media, such as Lowenstein–Jensen and Loeffler's serum are rendered sterile by heating at 80–85°C for half an hour on three successive days **(fractional sterilization).** This process is called **inspissation** and instrument used is called *inspissator*.
c. Water bath.

ii. Temperature at 100°C

a. **Boiling:** Boiling at 100°C for 10–30 minutes kills all vegetative spores and some bacterial spores. Sporing bacteria require prolonged periods of boiling. Therefore, it is not recommended for sterilization of instruments for surgical procedures.

b. Steam at atmospheric pressure at 100°C for 90 minutes. This can be provided by the traditional Koch and Arnold steamer (or by the multipurpose autoclave).
c. **Tyndallization:** An exposure of steam at 100°C for **20** minutes on three successive days is called **Tyndallization or intermittent sterilization.** This is a fractional method of sterilization. The instrument commonly used is Koch and Arnold steamer.

Principle: Vegetative cells and some spores are killed during the first heating and that the more resistant spores subsequently germinate and are killed during either the second or the third heating. Though generally adequate, this method may fail with spores of certain anaerobes and thermophiles.

Uses: This method is useful in sterilizing heat- sensitive culture media containing, such materials as carbohydrates, egg or serum, which are damaged by higher temperature of autoclave.

iii. Moist Heat at Temperature Above 100°C

Steam under pressure: Steam above 100°C or saturated steam is more efficient sterilizing agent than hot air.

Autoclave

Autoclaving is the process of sterilization by saturated steam under high pressure above 100°C. Steam sterilization is carried out in a pressure chamber called an **autoclave** (a device somewhat like a fancy pressure cooker).

Principle of autoclave

The principle of the autoclave or steam sterilizer is that water boils when its vapor pressure equals that of the surrounding atmosphere. When pressure inside a closed vessel increases, the temperature at which water boils also increases. Saturated steam has penetrative power and is a better sterilizing agent than dry heat.

Various components of autoclave

In its simplest form, the laboratory autoclave consists of a **vertical or horizontal cylinder of gunmetal or stainless steel**, in a supporting sheet iron case. **The lid or door** is fastened by screw clamps and made airtight by a suitable washer. The autoclave has on its lid or upper side a discharge tap for air and steam, a pressure gauge and a safety valve that can be set to blow off at any desired pressure. Heating is done by gas or electricity. The domestic pressure cooker serves as a miniature autoclave and may be used for sterilizing small articles in clinics and similar establishments.

Types of steam sterilizers

Several types of steam sterilizers are available. Even the domestic pressure cooker can be used as a sterilizer.

Procedure

1. **Water:** Sufficient water is put in the cylinder.
2. **Lid:** The lid is screwed tight with the discharge tap open and the safety valve is adjusted to the required pressure.
3. **Air removal:** The steam-air mixture is allowed to escape freely till all the air has been displaced.
4. The discharge tap is now closed.
5. **Holding period:** The steam pressure raises inside and when it reaches the desired set level (15 psi), the safety valve opens and the excess steam escapes. From this point, the holding period (15 minutes) is calculated.
6. **Autoclave cooling:** When the holding period is over, the heater is turned off and the autoclave allowed to cool.
7. **Air entry in the autoclave:** The discharge tap is opened slowly and air is allowed to enter the autoclave.
8. **Removal of articles:** The lid is now opened and the sterilized articles removed.

Note: Temperature: 121°C.

Chamber pressure

15 psi (per square inch)—these conditions are generally used. However, sterilization can also be done at higher temperatures, at 126°C (20 lbs/square inch) for 10 minutes or at 133°C (30 lbs/square inch) for 3 minutes.

Uses

i. For sterilizing culture media and other laboratory supplies, aqueous solutions, rubber material, dressing materials, gowns, dressing, linen, gloves, instruments, and pharmaceutical products.

ii. For all materials that are water containing, permeable or wettable and not liable to be damaged by the process.
iii. Particularly useful for materials which cannot withstand the higher temperature of hot air oven.

Sterilization controls
A. **Biological control (bacterial spores):** An envelope containing a filter paper strip impregnated with 10^6 spores of *Bacillus stearothermophilus* is placed with the load in the coolest and least accessible part of the autoclave chamber. No growth of *B. stearothermophilus* after sterilization is over and indicates proper sterilization.
B. **Chemical control:** A Browne's tube containing red solution changes to green when exposed to temperature of 121°C for 15 minutes in autoclave. It indicates proper sterilization.
C. Autoclave tapes
D. **Thermocouples:** May also be used which records the temperature by a potentiometer.

2. Filtration

Filtration is the principal method used in the laboratory for the sterilization of heat labile materials, e.g., sera, solutions of sugars, or antibiotics used for preparation of culture media.

Uses of Filtration
i. **Heat sensitive solutions:** For sterilization of pharmaceuticals, ophthalmic solutions, culture media, oils, antibiotics, and other heat sensitive solutions.
ii. **For separation of bacteriophages and bacterial toxins from bacteria.**
iii. **Isolation of organisms which are scanty in fluids.**
iv. **Concentration of bacteria from liquids.**
v. **For virus isolation.**

Types of Filters
i. **Earthenware filters:** These are manufactured in several different grades of porosity. The fluid to be sterilized is forced by suction or pressure from inside to outside or vice-versa.

ii. **Asbestos filters (Seitz filter):** They are made up of a disk of asbestos (magnesium trisilicate). It is supported on a perforated metal disk within a metal funnel. Filter disk is discarded after use.
iii. **Sintered glass filters:** They are prepared by size grading powdered glass followed by heating. The pore size can be controlled by the general particle size of the glass powder.
iv. **Membrane filters:** Membrane filters consist of a variety of polymeric materials, such as cellulose nitrate, cellulose diacetate, polycarbonate, and polyester. They are manufactured as disks from 13 to 293 mm diameter and with porosities from 0.015 to 12 mm.
v. Syringe filters
vi. Vacuum and "in-line" filters
vii. Pressure filtration
viii. Air filters

3. Radiation

Two types of radiations are used:
i. **Nonionizing:** Infrared and ultraviolet rays are of nonionizing type. The effectiveness of UV light as a lethal and mutagenic agent is closely correlated with its wavelength. It is most effectively absorbed by DNA and this infers with DNA replication. Ultraviolet radiation can be produced artificially by mercury vapor lamps.
Practical Applications
  a. To disinfect drinking water.
  b. **Disinfection of enclosed areas**—such as entryways, hospital wards, operating theaters, laboratories, and in ventilated safety cabinets in which dangerous microorganisms are being handled.
ii. **Ionizing radiation:** These include X-rays, γ (gamma) rays, and cosmic rays. These have very high penetrative power and are highly lethal to all cells including bacteria. Ionizing radiations damage the DNA by various mechanisms.
Applications
  i. For sterilization in pharmacy and medicine.
  ii. **Sterilization of packaged disposable articles**—such as plastic syringes, intravenous lines, catheters and gloves those are unable to withstand heat.

Cold sterilization: Since there is no appreciable increase in temperature in this method it is known as **cold sterilization**.

iii. **Use for antibiotics, hormones, sutures, and vaccines** and to prevent food spoilage.

Disinfection

Disinfection is used to destroy microorganisms. However, it does not destroy spores. The solutions used are called **disinfectants**, or possibly bactericidal solutions (the suffix "-cidal" is derived from a Latin word meaning "to kill"). These solutions are too strong for human skin to tolerate and are used only on inanimate objects. If a disinfectant solution comes in contact with human tissue, the tissue will feel "slippery". This is the first step of tissue breakdown. When using a disinfectant solution, use clean gloves to protect your skin.

B. Chemical Agents

Germicidal chemicals can be used to disinfect and, in some cases, sterilize **(Table 15.1)**.

TABLE 15.1: Chemical agents used in sterilization and disinfection.

Chemical Agent	Use
1. Surface-active agents	
i. Soaps and acid anionic detergents	Skin degerming and removal of debris.
ii. Acid-anionic detergents	Sanitizers in dairy and food-processing industries.
iii. Cationic detergents (quaternary ammonium compounds)	Antiseptic for skin, instruments, utensils, rubber goods.
2. Phenol and phenolics	
i. Phenol	Rarely used, except as a standard of comparison.
ii. Phenolics	Environmental surfaces, instruments, skin surfaces, and mucous membranes.
iii. Bisphenols	Disinfectant hand soaps and skin lotions.
3. Alcohols	Thermometers and other instruments; in swabbing the skin with alcohol before an injection, most of the disinfecting action probably comes from a simple wiping away (degerming) of dirt and some microbes.

Contd...

Contd...

Chemical agent	Use
4. Chemical food preservatives	
i. Organic acids	Sorbic acid and benzoic acid effective at low pH; parabens much used in. cosmetics, shampoos; calcium propionate used in bread.
ii. Nitrates/nitrites	Meat products such as ham. bacon. hot dogs, sausage.
5. Heavy metals and their compounds	Silver nitrate may be used to prevent gonorrheal ophthalmia neonatorum; mercurochrome disinfects skin and mucous membranes; copper sulfate is an algicide.
6. Halogens	Iodine is an effective antiseptic available as a tincture and an iodophor; chlorine gas is used to disinfect water; chlorine compounds are used to disinfect dairy equipment, eating utensils, household items, and glassware
7. Aldehydes	Glutaraldehyde (Cidex) is less irritating than formaldehyde and is used for disinfection of medical equipment.
8. Chemical sterilization	
i. Ethylene oxide and other gaseous sterilants	Mainly for sterilization of materials that would be damaged by heat.
ii. Plasma sterilization	Especially useful for tubular medical instruments.
iii. Supercritical fluids	Especially useful for sterilizing organic medical implants.
9. Peroxygens and other forms of oxygen	Contaminated surfaces; some deep wounds, in which they are very effective against oxygen-sensitive anaerobes.

Mechanisms of Action

The main modes of action are:
A. **Agents that damage the cell membrane**
  1. Surface active disinfectants
  2. Phenolic compounds
  3. Alcohols
B. **Agents that denature proteins**
  1. Acids and alkalis
  2. Alcohols

C. **Agents that modify functional groups of proteins and nucleic acids**
   1. Heavy metals and their compounds
   2. Oxidizing agents
      - Halogens
      - Hydrogen peroxide
   3. Dyes
      - Aniline dyes
      - Acridine dyes
   4. Alkylating agents
      - Aldehydes: Formaldehyde, glutaraldehyde
      - Ethylene oxide

Chemical Agents

1. Surface-active Agents

Substances that alter the energy relationships at interfaces, producing a reduction of surface or interfacial tension, are referred to as **surface-active agents or surfactants**.

Classification: These surfactants are classified into cationic, anionic, nonionic and ampholytic (amphoteric). Of these, the cationic and anionic compounds have been the most useful antibacterial agents.

A. **Cationic agents: Quaternary ammonium compounds (quats)** include cetrimide (cetavlon), benzalkonium chloride (Zephiran, a brand name) and cetylpyridinium chloride (Cepacol, a brand name).
B. **Anionic agents:** These include soap and fatty acids.
C. **Ampholytic (amphoteric) compounds** known as "**Tego**" compounds.

2. Phenols and Phenolics

Phenol derivatives: Certain phenol derivatives, such as **cresol, chlorhexidine, chloroxylenol,** and **hexachlorophene** are commonly used as antiseptics.
1. **Cresols:** Cresols is sold under the trade names of *Lysol* and *Creolin*. "**White fluids**" such as Lysol are most commonly used for sterilization of infected glass wares, cleaning floors, disinfection of excreta.

2. **Chlorhexidine: Savlon (chlorhexidine and cetrimide)** is widely used in wounds, preoperative disinfection of skin, as bladder irrigant, etc. However, contact with the eyes can cause damage.
3. **Chloroxylenol:** It is an active ingredient of Dettol.
4. **Hexachlorophene:** Used for surgical and hospital microbial control procedures.

3. Alcohols

Ethyl alcohol (ethanol) and **isopropyl alcohol** are the most frequently used. They must be used at a concentration of 60–70% in water to be effective. They are most frequently used as skin disinfectants and act by **denaturing bacterial proteins.**

4. Chemical Food Preservatives
 i. Organic acids
 ii. Nitrates/nitrites

5. Heavy Metals

For many years the ions of heavy metals, such as **mercury, silver, arsenic, zinc, and copper** were used as germicides.

6. Halogens

Chlorine and **iodine** are among the most useful disinfectants.
a. **Iodine**: Iodine compounds are the most effective halogens available for disinfection.
   Uses
   i. Skin disinfectant
   ii. **Iodophor Povidone-iodine (betadine)** for wounds and *Wescodyne* for skin and laboratory disinfection are some popular brands.
b. **Chlorine:** In addition to **chlorine** itself, there are three types of chlorine compound **hypochlorites, inorganic, and organic chloramines.** The disinfectant action of all chlorine compounds is due to the liberation of free chlorine.
   Uses: The usual disinfectant for water supplies, swimming pools, dairy, and food industries.
c. **Hypochlorites: Bleaching powder or hypochlorite solution** is the most widely used for human immunodeficiency virus (HIV) infected material.
   Chloramines are used as antiseptics for dressing wounds.

Chapter 15: Sterilization and Disinfection

7. Aldehydes

The lethal effects of aldehydes (formaldehyde and glutaraldehyde) and ethylene dioxide result from their alkylating action on proteins.

i. **Formaldehyde:** Formaldehyde is employed in the liquid and vapor states. Exposure of skin or mucus membranes to formaldehyde can be toxic and the gas is irritant and toxic when inhaled.

Uses
   a. **Formalin:**
      i. Used for preserving fresh tissues.
      ii. Formalin has been used to inactivate viruses in the **preparation of vaccines**.
   b. **Formaldehyde:**
      i. It is used to preserve anatomical specimens
      ii. For destroying anthrax spores in hair
      iii. As an antiseptic mouthwash
      iv. For the disinfection of membranes in dialysis equipment
      v. A preservative in hair shampoos
   c. **Formaldehyde gas:**
      i. Used for sterilizing instruments, heat sensitive catheters and for fumigating wards, sick rooms and laboratories.
      ii. Clothing, bedding, furniture, and books can be satisfactorily disinfected under properly controlled conditions.

ii. **Glutaraldehyde:** This has an action similar to formaldehyde. It is used as 2% buffered solution. It can be used for delicate instruments having lenses. It is available commercially as "cidex".

Uses
   a. **Cold sterilant:** It has been used increasingly as a **cold sterilant** for **surgical instruments,** such as cystoscopes, endoscopes, and bronchoscope.
   b. Used safely to sterilize corrugated rubber anesthetic tubes and face masks, plastic endotracheal tubes, metal instruments, and polythene tubing.

8. Chemical Sterilization

Sterilization with liquid chemicals is possible, but even sporicidal chemicals, such as glutaraldehyde are usually not considered to be practical sterilants. However, the gaseous chemosterilants are frequently used as substitutes for physical sterilization processes.

Their application requires a closed chamber similar to a steam autoclave. Probably the most familiar example is *ethylene oxide:*
1. ***Ethylene oxide:*** It is highly inflammable and, in concentrations in air >3%, highly explosive.
   Uses
   a. **Sterilization of articles liable to be damaged by heat:** It is especially used for sterilizing heart-lung machines, respirators, sutures, dental equipment, books, and clothing.
   b. **Sterilization of a wide range of materials**— such as glass, metal and paper surfaces, clothing, plastics, soil, some foods, and tobacco.

   Chlorine dioxide is a short-lived gas has been used to fumigate enclosed building areas contaminated with endospores of anthrax.
2. ***Plasma sterilization:*** Plasma is a state of matter in which a gas is excited, in this case by an electromagnetic field, to make a mixture of nuclei with assorted electrical charges and free electrons. Plasma sterilization is a reliable method to sterilizing metal or plastic surgical instruments used for many newer procedures in arthroscopic or laparoscopic surgery.

   Advantage: It requires only low temperatures, but it is relatively expensive.
3. ***Supercritical fluids***: The use of supercritical fluids in sterilization combines chemical and physical methods. When carbon dioxide is compressed into a "supercritical" state, it has properties of both a liquid (with increased solubility) and a gas (with a lowered surface tension). Supercritical carbon dioxide has more recently been used to decontaminate medical implants, such as bone, tendons, or ligaments taken from donor patients.

9. Peroxygens and Other Forms of Oxygen

Peroxygens are a group of oxidizing agents that includes hydrogen peroxide and peracetic acid.
   i. **Hydrogen peroxide:** It is an antiseptic found in many household medicine cabinets and in hospital supply rooms. The food industry is increasing its use of hydrogen peroxide for aseptic packaging. Hydrogen peroxide is used to disinfect plastic implants, contact lenses, and surgical prosthesis.

ii. **Peracetic acid (peroxyacetic acid or PAA):** It is one of the most effective liquid chemical sporicides available and can be used as a sterilant. Its mode of action is similar to that of hydrogen peroxide.

   Applications: Disinfection of food-processing and medical equipment, especially endoscopes.

   Other oxidizing agents include *benzoyl peroxide*, which is probably most familiar as the main ingredient in over-the-counter medications for acne.

iii. ***Ozone (O_3)*** is a highly reactive form of oxygen that is generated by passing oxygen through high-voltage electrical discharges. Ozone is often used to supplement chlorine in the disinfection of water because it helps neutralize tastes and odors. Although ozone is a more effective killing agent than chlorine, its residual activity is difficult to maintain in water.

Categories of Disinfectant

See **Box 15.2.**

Disinfection Guidelines

1. Surfaces and items to disinfect floors, door knobs, window handles, buttons, switches, furniture surfaces, telephones, intercoms, trash cans, sinks, toilets, bath tubs, faucets, shower heads, floor drains, ventilators, computers, keyboards, fans, etc.
2. **Tools and equipment:** Alcohol or bleach (0.05% sodium hypochlorite), towels, rubber gloves and masks.
3. **Disinfection procedures:**
   a. Start with wiping clean the less soiled surfaces.
   b. Towels should be soaked in bleach before use.
   c. Rinse articles and surfaces with water and wipe dry 10 minutes after disinfection.
   d. Diluted bleach can be used to disinfect toilets.
   e. Do not flush large amounts or highly concentrated bleach down the toilet to keep sewage treatment plant running smoothly. Wear a mask and rubber gloves while using bleach.

> **Box 15.2:** Categories of disinfectant.

1. **High-level disinfection**: A germicide that kills all microbial pathogens except large numbers of bacterial spores. High-level disinfection can generally approach sterilization in effectiveness, whereas spore forms can survive intermediate-level disinfection, and many microbes can remain viable when exposed to low-level disinfection. High-level disinfectants are used for items involved with invasive procedures that cannot withstand sterilization procedures (e.g., certain types of endoscopes, surgical instruments with plastic or other components that cannot be autoclaved).
   Examples:
   – Treatment with moist heat
   – Use of liquids, such as glutaraldehyde, hydrogen peroxide, peracetic acid, chlorine dioxide, and other chlorine compounds.
2. **Intermediate-level disinfectants:** A germicide that kills all microbial pathogens except bacterial endospores. Intermediate-level disinfectants are used to clean surfaces or instruments in which contamination with bacterial spores and other highly resilient organisms is unlikely. These include flexible fiber-optic endoscopes, laryngoscopes, vaginal specula, anesthesia breathing circuits, and other items. These have been referred to as semicritical instruments and devices.
   Examples: Alcohols, iodophor compounds, phenolic compounds.
3. **Low-level disinfectants**: A germicide that kills most vegetative bacteria and lipid-enveloped and medium-size viruses. Low-level disinfectants are used to treat noncritical instruments and devices, such as blood pressure cuffs, electrocardiogram electrodes, and stethoscopes. They do not penetrate through mucosal surfaces or into sterile tissues although, these items come into contact with patients.
   Example: Quaternary ammonium compounds.

RECOMMENDED CONCENTRATIONS OF DISINFECTANTS COMMONLY USED IN THE HOSPITALS (TABLE 15.2)

TABLE 15.2: List the recommended concentrations of disinfectants commonly used in the hospitals.

Disinfectant	Concentration
Betadine (iodophor)	2%
Bleaching powder (calcium hypochlorite)	14 g in 1 L of water
Dettol (chloroxylenol)	4%
Ethyl alcohol	70%
Glutaraldehyde	2%
Lysol	2.5%
Savlon (chlorhexidine and cetrimide)	2%, 5%
Sodium hypochlorite	1%, 0.1%

■ CLEANING

Cleaning is the removal of foreign materials, such as soil and organic material, from objects. Generally, cleaning involves use of water and mechanical action with or without detergents. When an object comes in contact with infectious or potentially infectious material, the object is contaminated. If the object is disposable, it is usually discarded unless formal policies and procedures are in place for reprocessing the object. It is necessary to thoroughly clean reusable objects and then either disinfect or sterilize them before reuse.

Environmental Cleaning

The term "environmental cleaning" (EC) refers broadly to the organized processes employed by hospitals for cleaning, disinfecting, and monitoring. Environmental cleaning is a fundamental principle of preventing infection in the hospital setting. Both porous surfaces (e.g., mattresses) and nonporous surfaces (e.g., bed rails) in patient rooms are highly susceptible to bacterial contamination with dangerous pathogens, including *Clostridium difficile*, and antibiotic-resistant organisms, such as methicillin-resistant *Staphylococcus aureus* (MRSA), vancomycin-resistant *enterococci* (VRE), and multiple species of *Acinetobacter* (*Acinetobacter* spp). Hard, nonporous surfaces, which include common items, such as furniture, bed rails, and medical equipment, as well as fixed spaces such as floors and bathroom facilities, form part of the environmental reservoir that can lead to significant microbial contamination. Appropriate cleaning of these surfaces is an important part of an overall strategy to reduce the risk of healthcare-associated infections (HAIs).

A wide variety of cleaning agents and disinfection technologies are commercially available, each with potential benefits and disadvantages. Additionally, hospitals often monitor the quality of room cleaning and disinfection to ensure that surfaces have been treated appropriately. Several monitoring strategies exist, which range from simple visual inspection, to microbiologic testing of surface contamination, to technologic innovations that measure the adequacy of surface cleaning. As the variety of options for cleaning, disinfecting, and monitoring grow, hospitals are faced with many choices, but limited evidence exists on the comparative effectiveness of these interventions, especially related to HAI rates within the hospital.

Equipment Cleaning

When cleaning equipment, i.e., soiled by organic material, such as blood, fecal matter, mucus, or pus, put on a mask and protective eyewear or goggles (or a face shield) and waterproof gloves. These barriers provide protection from infectious organisms (as discussed earlier). You will need a stiff bristled brush and detergent or soap for cleaning. The following steps ensure that an object is clean:

1. Rinse a contaminated object or article with cold running water to remove organic material. Hot water causes the protein in organic material to coagulate and stick to objects, making removal difficult.
2. After rinsing, wash the object with soap and warm water. Soap or detergent reduces the surface tension of water and emulsifies dirt and remaining material. Rinse the object thoroughly to remove the emulsified dirt.
3. Use a brush to remove dirt or material in grooves or seams. Friction dislodges contaminated material for easy removal. Open any hinged items for cleaning.
4. Rinse the object in warm water.
5. Dry the object and prepare it for disinfection or sterilization, if indicated by the intended use of the item.
6. Consider the brush, the gloves, and the sink in which the equipment is cleaned contaminated and make sure it is cleaned and dried per hospital protocol.

■ ASEPSIS

Asepsis is absence of pathogenic microorganisms. It is divided into two categories—medical and surgical:

1. **Medical asepsis (clean technique):** It consists of techniques that inhibit the growth and spread of pathogenic microorganisms. Medical asepsis is also known as **clean technique** and is used in many daily activities. They include hand washing, bathing, cleaning environment, gloving, gowning, wearing masks, hair and shoe covers, disinfecting articles, and use of antiseptics changing patients' bed linen. You follow principles of medical asepsis in the home, for instance, with the common practice of washing your hands before preparing food.
2. **Surgical asepsis (sterile technique):** It destroys all microorganisms and their **spores** (the reproductive cell of some microorganisms,

such as fungi or protozoa). Surgical asepsis is known as **sterile technique** and is used in specialized areas or skills, such as care of surgical wounds, urinary catheter insertion, invasive procedures, and surgery.

■ SPAULDING'S CLASSIFICATION

Spaulding's classification was proposed by Earle H Spaulding in 1939, and it is the guideline that should determine the disinfection or sterilization method that should be chosen according to the medical instrument (**Table 15.3**).

Critical items: Instruments that touch places where no single microorganism should exist are critical items, e.g., a surgical instrument. These must be sterilized unconditionally.

TABLE 15.3: Spaulding's classification of medical equipment/devices and required level of processing/reprocessing.

Classification	Definition	Level of processing/ reprocessing	Examples
Critical Equipment/ device	Equipment/device that enters sterile tissues, including the vascular system	Cleaning followed by sterilization	❖ Surgical instruments ❖ Implants ❖ Biopsy instruments ❖ Foot care equipment ❖ Eye and dental equipment
Semicritical equipment/ device	Equipment/device that comes in contact with non-intact skin or mucous membranes but does not penetrate them	❖ Cleaning followed by high-level ❖ Disinfection (as a minimum) ❖ Sterilization is preferred	❖ Respiratory therapy equipment ❖ Anesthesia equipment ❖ Tonometer
Noncritical equipment/ device	Equipment/device that touches only intact skin and not mucous membranes, or does not directly touch the client/ patient/resident	❖ Cleaning followed by low-level ❖ Disinfection (in some cases, cleaning alone is acceptable)	❖ ECG machines ❖ Oximeters ❖ Bedpans, urinals, commodes

Semicritical items: Instruments that contact incised skin or mucous membranes are semicritical items, e.g., endoscopes and anesthesia equipment. These should undergo high-level disinfection.

Noncritical items: Instruments that touch intact skin are noncritical items, e.g., fomites. These require low-level disinfection.

KEY POINTS

- Sterilization is the process by which an article, surface, or medium is freed of all living microorganisms either in the vegetative or spore state
- Disinfection is the killing, inhibition, or removal of microorganisms that may cause disease.
- Cleaning is the removal of foreign materials, such as soil and organic material, from objects.
- The term "environmental cleaning" refers broadly to the organized processes employed by hospitals for cleaning, disinfecting, and monitoring.
- **Methods of sterilization and disinfection:**
  - Physical agents: Heat (dry heat, moist heat); filtration, radiation, ultrasonic and sonic vibrations.
  - Chemical agents:
    1. **Surface-active agents:**
       a. Cationic agents
       b. Anionic agents
       c. Ampholytic (amphoteric) agents
    2. **Phenol and phenolics:** Certain phenol derivatives such as **cresol, chlorhexidine, chloroxylenol,** and **hexachlorophene** are commonly used as antiseptics.
    3. **Alcohols:** Ethyl alcohol (ethanol) and isopropyl alcohol are the most frequently used.
    4. **Chemical food preservatives**
    5. **Heavy metals:** Mercuric chloride, silver nitrate
    6. **Halogens:**
       a. Iodine
       b. Chlorine
       c. Hypochlorites

7. **Aldehydes:** The lethal effects of aldehydes (formaldehyde and glutaraldehyde) and ethylene dioxide result from their alkylating action on proteins.
8. **Chemical sterilization:**
     i. Ethylene oxide and other gaseous sterilants
     ii. Plasma sterilization
     iii. Supercritical fluids
9. **Peroxygens and other forms of oxygen**

IMPORTANT QUESTIONS

1. Define sterilization and disinfection. Classify the various agents used in sterilization.
2. Define the terms sterilization, disinfection and cleaning. Name various agents used for sterilization and disinfection.
3. Define sterilization. Classify the methods of sterilization.
4. Write short notes on:
   a. Spaulding's classification
   b. Environment cleaning
   c. Equipment cleaning
5. Name various types of disinfectants and discuss the role of halogens in chemical disinfection.
6. Give an account of testing antimicrobial potency of disinfectants and antiseptics.
7. Write short notes on:
   a. Phenols as disinfectants
   b. Halogens as disinfectants
   c. Aldehydes as disinfectants
   d. Alcohols as disinfectants
   e. Vapor-phase disinfectants or gaseous sterilization
   f. Surface active disinfectants
   g. Quaternary ammonium compounds
   h. Oxidizing agents

MULTIPLE CHOICE QUESTIONS (MCQs)

1. **The holder method of pasteurization is not effective against:**
   a. *Escherichia coli*
   b. *Coxiella burnetii*
   c. *Staphylococcus aureus*
   d. *Salmonella typhi*

2. The bacterial spore that is most frequently used as indicator of sterilization by hot air oven is:
   a. *Bacillus subtilis*
   b. *Clostridium tetani*
   c. *Bacillus pumilus*
   d. *Bacillus globigii*
3. Which of the following does not kill endospores?
   a. Autoclaving
   b. Hot air sterilization
   c. Pasteurization
   d. None of the above
4. Sterilization at 100°C for 20 minutes on three successive days is known as:
   a. Tyndallization
   b. Inspissation
   c. Pasteurization
   d. Vaccine bath
5. Which bacterial spores are used as sterilization control in autoclave?
   a. *Bacillus cereus*
   b. *Bacillus stearothermophilus*
   c. *Clostridium perfringens*
   d. *Pseudomonas aeruginosa*
6. Autoclave is not useful for sterilization of:
   a. Disposable plastic petri dishes
   b. Surgical dressings
   c. Metallic instruments
   d. Liquid paraffin
7. Which of the following is most effective for sterilizing mattresses and petri dishes?
   a. Chlorine
   b. Autoclaving
   c. Ethylene oxide
   d. Glutaraldehyde
8. Which one of these disinfectants does not act by disrupting the plasma membrane?
   a. Phenolics
   b. Ethylene oxide
   c. Halogens
   d. Phenol
9. Ionizing radiation can be used for sterilization of:
   a. Plastic syringes
   b. Gloves
   c. Catheters
   d. All of the above
10. The most widely used disinfectant for human immunodeficiency virus (HIV) infected material is:
    a. Phenol
    b. Lysol
    c. Hypochlorite solution
    d. Silver nitrate
11. Glutaraldehyde is used as a cold sterilant for sterilization of:
    a. Cystoscopes
    b. Endoscopes
    c. Bronchoscope
    d. All of the above
12. All the following statements are true for ethylene oxide, *except*:
    a. It diffuses through many types of porous materials.
    b. It is used for sterilizing heart-lung machines, respirators, books, and clothing.

c. It is used for sterilizing glass, metal and paper surfaces, clothing, plastics, and some foods.
d. It is suitable for fumigating rooms.
13. Which test is used to simulate the natural conditions under which the disinfectants are used in the hospitals?
   a. Kelsey–Sykes capacity test
   b. Rideal–Walker test
   c. In-use test
   d. Chick–Martin test

ANSWERS

1. b	2. a	3. C	4. a	5. b	6. d
7. c	8. c	9. d	10. c	11. d	12. d
13. a					

CHAPTER 16

Antimicrobial Chemotherapy

Learning Objectives

After reading and studying this chapter, you should be able to:
- Describe mechanism of action of antibacterial drugs.
- Describe mechanism of drug resistance.
- List cephalosporins of first, second, third, and fourth generation.

■ INTRODUCTION

Antimicrobial Agent

Antimicrobial agent is a chemical substance inhibiting the growth or causing the death of a microorganism.

Antibiotic

Antibiotic as originally defined was a chemical substance produced by various species of microorganisms that was capable of inhibiting the growth or causing death of other microorganisms in low concentration. However, with the advent of synthetic methods, this definition has been modified.

Chemotherapeutic Agents

Chemotherapeutic agents are the chemical substances used to kill or inhibit the growth of microorganisms already established in the tissues of the body. Nowadays, the term ***antibiotic*** is used loosely to describe agents (mainly, but not exclusively, antibacterial agents) used to treat systemic infection.

Antimicrobial agent (AMA): It would be more meaningful to use the term **AMA** to designate synthetic as well as naturally obtained drugs that attenuate microorganisms.

Antiseptics or disinfectants: Antimicrobial substances that are too toxic to be used other than in topical therapy or for environmental decontamination are referred to as *antiseptics* or *disinfectants*.

■ ANTIBACTERIAL AGENTS

The principal types of antibacterial agents are listed in **Table 15.1**. These have been grouped according to their site of action.

TABLE 15.1: Mechanisms of antibacterial drug action.

1. **Inhibitors of bacterial cell wall synthesis**
    - Penicillins
    - Cephalosporins
    - Vancomycin
    - Bacitracin
    - Cycloserine
    - Fosfomycin
2. **Inhibitors of bacterial cytoplasmic membrane function**
    - Polymyxins
    - Gramicidin
    - Tyrocidine
3. **Inhibition of bacterial nucleic acid synthesis**
    - Quinolones
    - Rifamycins
    - Nitroimidazoles
    - Nitrofurans
    - Novobiocin
4. **Inhibition of bacterial protein synthesis**
    - Aminoglycosides
    - Chloramphenicol
    - Tetracyclines
    - Macrolides
    - Lincosamides
    - Fusidic acid
    - Streptogramins
    - Mupirocins
5. **Metabolic antagonism**
    - Sulfonamides
    - Trimethoprim
    - Dapsone
    - Isoniazid

■ MECHANISMS OF ACTION OF ANTIBACTERIAL DRUGS

Mechanisms of action of antibacterial agents can be placed under the headings:
1. Inhibition of bacterial cell wall synthesis
2. Inhibition of bacterial cytoplasmic membrane function
3. Inhibition of bacterial nucleic acid synthesis
4. Inhibition of bacterial protein synthesis

Inhibition of Bacterial Cell Wall Synthesis

The antibiotics which inhibit cell wall synthesis are β-lactam antibiotics (penicillins and cephalosporins), glycopeptides, bacitracin, cycloserine, fosfomycin and isoniazid.

β-lactam Agents

This group includes penicillins, cephalosporins and other compounds that feature a β-lactam ring in their structure.

Penicillins

Each member of the family of penicillins shares a common basic structure. Penicillins are a group of antimicrobial substances, all of which possess a common chemical nucleus (6-aminopenicillanic acid) which contains a β-lactam ring essential to their biologic activity.

Resistance to Penicillin

Resistance to penicillin may be due to:
  i. Production of penicillin-destroying enzymes (β-lactamases).
  ii. Impermeability of cell envelope.
  iii. Alteration or lack of penicillin receptors.
  iv. Failure of activation of autolytic enzymes in the cell wall, e.g., in staphylococci.
  v. Cell-wall deficient (L) forms or mycoplasmas, which do not synthesize peptidoglycan.

Cephalosporins

Cephalosporins are a family of antibiotics originally isolated in 1948 from the fungus *Cephalosporium,* and their β-lactam structure is very similar to that of the penicillins. They are grouped as the first-, second-, third-, and fourth generation cephalosporins. These include cephalexin and cephradine (first generation), cefaclor and cefprozil (second generation), cefixime and ceftibuten (third generation), and cefepime (fourth generation). The later generations are generally more effective against gram-negative bacteria and are less susceptible to destruction by β-lactamases.

Other β-lactam Antibiotics

Various agents with diverse properties share the structural feature of a β-lactam ring with penicillins and cephalosporins. Two other groups of β-lactam drugs, **carbapenems** and **monobactams**, are very resistant to β-lactamases.

Glycopeptides

Two glycopeptides, vancomycin and teicoplanin, are in clinical use. They are mainly used in serious infections with staphylococci and enterococci that are resistant to other drugs.

Inhibition of Bacterial Cytoplasmic Membrane Function

Only polymyxins have been regularly used systemically among membrane active agents used in human medicine. Two members of the family are in therapeutic use—polymyxin B and colistin (polymyxin E).

Polymyxin B and colistin (polymyxin E) exhibit potent antipseudomonal activity, but toxicity has limited their usefulness, except in topical preparations and bowel decontamination regimens.

Inhibitors of Nucleic Acid Synthesis

Quinolones

The quinolones are synthetic drugs that contain the 4-quinolone ring. The first quinolone, nalidixic acid was synthesized in 1962. **Nalidixic acid and its early congeners** are narrow-spectrum agents active only against gram-negative bacteria.

Newer quinolones such as ciprofloxacin, norfloxacin, ofloxacin, pefloxacin and lomefloxacin are broad spectrum quinolones. These have been successfully used in a wide variety of infections, but resistance is becoming more prevalent.

Rifamycins

This group of antibiotics is characterized by excellent activity against mycobacteria, although other bacteria are also susceptible. Staphylococci in particular are exquisitely sensitive. Rifampicin and rifabutin are most widely used.

Nitroimidazoles

The representative of the group most commonly used clinically is metronidazole, but similar derivatives include tinidazole, ornidazole and nimorazole. They are primarily antiprotozoal agents, but they exhibit potent activity against anaerobic bacteria.

Nitrofurans

These include:
- **Nitrofurantoin**—an agent used exclusively in urinary tract infection.
- **Furazolidone**—is used in enteric infections.

Novobiocin

It is quite active against staphylococci and streptococci, but is no longer favored because of problems of resistance and toxicity. *Staphylococcus saprophyticus* is novobiocin resistant.

Inhibition of Bacterial Protein Synthesis

Several types of antibacterial drugs inhibit prokaryotic protein synthesis. Of these, only the aminoglycosides are bactericidal; the others are all bacteriostatic. Two classes of drugs that have recently been approved for use are the oxazolidinones and the streptogramins. A synergistic combination of two streptogramins is bactericidal against some organisms.

Chloramphenicol: Use of chloramphenicol has been limited to typhoid fever, meningitis and a few other clinical indications.

Tetracyclines: Tetracyclines are broad-spectrum agents with important activity against chlamydiae, rickettsiae, mycoplasmas and, surprisingly, malaria parasites, as well as most conventional

Metabolic Antagonism

Sulfonamides and diaminopyrimidines: They are now little used alone, but the combination of sulfamethoxazole with trimethoprim (cotrimoxazole) is still widely used.

■ RESISTANCE TO ANTIMICROBIAL DRUGS

The spread of drug-resistant pathogens is one of the most serious threats to the successful treatment of microbial disease.

Mechanisms of Drug Resistance

The most common mechanisms of acquired antimicrobial resistance are:
1. Drug-inactivating enzymes:
   Penicillinase: The best-known example is the hydrolysis of the β-lactam ring of many penicillins by the enzyme penicillinase.
2. Alteration in the target molecule:
   Examples: Alterations in the penicillin-binding proteins prevent β-lactam drugs from binding to them.
3. Decreased uptake of the drug
4. Increased elimination of the drug.

KEY POINTS

- **Antibiotic** as originally defined was a chemical substance produced by various species of microorganisms that was capable of inhibiting the growth or causing death of other microorganisms in low concentration.
- **Chemotherapeutic agents** are the chemical substances used to kill or inhibit the growth of microorganisms already established in the tissues of the body.

IMPORTANT QUESTIONS

1. Define the terms antimicrobial agent, chemotherapeutic agent, and antibiotics. Name various mechanisms of action of antibiotics giving examples.
2. Write short notes on:
   a. Cephalosporins
   b. Quinolones

MULTIPLE CHOICE QUESTIONS (MCQs)

1. Which of the following antibiotics act/s by inhibiting cell wall synthesis?
   a. Penicillins
   b. Vancomycin
   c. Bacitracin
   d. All of the above
2. Which of the following antibiotics acts by inhibiting cytoplasmic membrane?
   a. Polymyxin
   b. Thyrocidine
   c. Gramicidin
   d. All of the above
3. Which antibiotic/s act/s by inhibiting bacterial nucleic acid synthesis?
   a. Quinolones
   b. Novobiocin
   c. Nitrofurans
   d. All of the above
4. Which of the following antibiotics act/s by inhibiting bacterial protein synthesis?
   a. Aminoglycosides
   b. Tetracycline
   c. Macrolides
   d. All of the above
5. Which antibiotic/s act/s as metabolic antagonists for their action?
   a. Sulfones
   b. Trimethoprim
   c. Isoniazid
   d. All of the above
6. What is the genetic basis of drug resistance in *Mycobacterium tuberculosis*?
   a. Transformation
   b. Transduction
   c. Mutation
   d. Conjugation
7. *Staphylococcus aureus* acquire drug resistance by:
   a. Transformation
   b. Transduction
   c. Mutation
   d. Conjugation

ANSWERS

1. d   2. d   3. d   4. d   5. d   6. c
7. b

CHAPTER 17

Biomedical Waste Management

Learning Objectives

After reading and studying this chapter, you should be able to:
* Define and classify biomedical waste.
* Describe various methods of treatment and disposal technologies for healthcare waste.
* Describe laws related to biomedical waste management in India.
* Describe laundry management process and infection control and prevention.

■ INTRODUCTION

Hospitals regularly generate waste, which may be a potential health hazard to healthcare workers (HCWs), the general public, and the environment. Therefore, adequate management and disposal of waste is essential.

Agents, which are associated with laboratory acquired infections: Most common agents, which are associated with laboratory acquired infections include hepatitis B virus, *Coccidioides immitis, Bacillus anthracis, Brucella* species, *Mycobacterium tuberculosis, Francisella tularensis,* and *Shigella* species.

Definition of Biomedical Waste

According to Biomedical waste (Management and Handling) Rules, 1998 of India, "Biomedical waste (BMW)" means any waste, which is generated during the diagnosis, treatment, or immunization of human beings or animals or in research activities pertaining there to or in the production or testing of biologicals.

Between 75 and 90% of the waste produced by the healthcare providers is **nonrisk or "general"** healthcare waste, comparable to domestic waste. The remaining 10–25% healthcare waste is regarded as **hazardous** and may create a variety of health risk.

Infectious wastes include all those medical wastes, which have the potential to transmit viral, bacterial, or parasitic diseases. It includes both human and animal infectious waste and waste generated in laboratories, and veterinary practice.

Infectious waste is hazardous in nature. Any waste with a potential to pose a threat to human health and life is called **hazardous waste**.

Non-infectious hazardous waste may be chemical (toxic, corrosive, inflammable, reactive, and otherwise injurious), radioactive, and pharmacological (surplus or time expired drugs).

Categories of Biomedical Waste

The categories and types of BMW are given in **Box 17.1**.

Waste Segregation

The BMW should be segregated into containers/bags at the point of generation of the waste.

Collection bags: The BMW should be segregated into containers/bags at the point of generation of the waste. Solid waste is collected in leak-resistant heavy-duty bags. Colored bags made of nonchlorinated plastic with biohazard sign and labels mentioning date and details of the waste are to be used. The bags are tied tightly after they are three-fourths full. Waste should be segregated in bags of different colors to facilitate appropriate treatment and disposal **(Table 17.1)**.

Box 17.1: Categories of biomedical waste and types of waste.

- **Yellow:** For human anatomical waste, animal anatomical waste, soiled waste, expired or discarded medicines, chemical waste, chemical liquid waste, discarded contaminated beddings and microbiology, biotechnology, and other clinical waste
- **Red:** For contaminated plastic waste
- **White (translucent):** For **waste sharps including metals**
- **Blue:** For (a) **Glassware;** (b) **Metallic body implants**

Types of bags or containers used for BMW **(Table 17.1)**:
A. Yellow bags
B. Red bags
C. White (translucent)
D. Blue

Treatment and Disposal Technologies for Healthcare Waste (Table 17.1)

Waste Treatment

Following techniques are used for the treatment of infected material:

1. Incineration

Incineration is a high-temperature dry oxidation process that reduces organic and combustible waste to inorganic incombustible matter and results in a very significant reduction of waste—volume and weight. This is a safe method of treating large solid infectious waste, particularly anatomy waste, and amputated limbs, animal carcasses and the like. The incinerator subjects them to very high heat, converting them to ash, which would be only about a tenth of original volume. However, it is expensive and is generally used only by very large establishments.

Types of Incinerators

Three basic kinds of incineration technology are of interest for treating healthcare waste:
1. Double-chamber pyrolytic incinerators, which may be especially designed to burn infectious healthcare waste.
2. Single-chamber furnaces with static grate, which should be used only if pyrolytic incinerators are not affordable; and
3. Rotary kilns operating at high temperatures are capable of causing decomposition of genotoxic substances and heat-resistant chemicals.

Double Chambered Incineration

Incinerators should be installed at appropriate location, to avoid nuisance to patients and neighborhood. An incinerator should consist of two chambers, primary and secondary.

The temperature of primary chamber should be 750–850°C while the temperature in the secondary chamber should be 1,000–1,100°C. Waste is burnt in one chamber (primary chamber) at 800°C. Combustion of gases emitted from the first chamber, occurs in the second or secondary chamber, which has a high temperature of 1,000°C. The negative pressure is maintained inside the incinerator by the system, thereby forcing the end-gases out of the chimney.

TABLE 17.1: Biomedical wastes categories and their segregation, collection, treatment, processing, and disposal options.

		Part-I	
Category	Type of waste	Types of bag or container to be used	Treatment and disposal options
(1)	(2)	(3)	(4)
Yellow	a. **Human anatomical waste:** Human tissues, organs, body parts, and fetus below the viability period (as per the Medical Termination of Pregnancy Act 1971, amended from time to time)	Yellow colored nonchlorinated plastic bags	Incineration or plasma pyrolysis or deep burial*
	b. **Animal anatomical waste:** Experimental animal carcasses, body parts, organs, tissues, including the waste generated from animals used in experiments or testing in veterinary hospitals or colleges or animal houses		
	c. **Soiled waste:** Items contaminated with blood, body fluids, such as dressings, plaster casts, cotton swabs, and bags containing residual or discarded blood and blood components		Incineration or plasma pyrolysis or deep burial.* In absence of above facilities, autoclaving or microwaving/ hydroclaving followed by shredding or mutilation or combination of sterilization and shredding. Treated waste to be sent for energy recovery.

Contd...

Contd...

Category (1)	Type of waste (2)	Types of bag or container to be used (3)	Treatment and disposal options (4)
	d. **Expired or discarded medicines:** Pharmaceutical waste like antibiotics, cytotoxic drugs including all items contaminated with cytotoxic drugs along with glass or plastic ampoules, vials, etc.	Yellow-colored nonchlorinated plastic bags or containers	Expired cytotoxic drugs and items contaminated with cytotoxic drugs to be returned back to the manufacturer or supplier for incineration at temperature >1,200°C or to common biomedical waste treatment facility or hazardous waste treatment, storage, and disposal facility for incineration at >1,200°C or encapsulation or plasma pyrolysis at >1,200°C. All other discarded medicines shall be either sent back to manufacturer or disposed by incineration
	e. **Chemical waste:** Chemicals used in production of biological and used or discarded disinfectants	Yellow colored containers or nonchlorinated plastic bags	Disposed of by incineration or plasma pyrolysis or encapsulation in hazardous waste treatment, storage, and disposal facility
	f. **Chemical liquid waste:** Liquid waste generated due to the use of chemicals in production of biological and used or discarded disinfectants, silver X-ray film developing liquid, discarded formalin, infected secretions, aspirated body fluids, liquid from laboratories and floor washings, cleaning, house keeping, and disinfecting activities, etc.	Separate collection system leading to effluent treatment system	After resource recovery, the chemical liquid waste shall be pretreated before mixing with other wastewater. The combined discharge shall conform to the discharge norms given in Schedule-III.

Contd...

Contd...

Category (1)	Type of waste (2)	Types of bag or container to be used (3)	Treatment and disposal options (4)
	g. Discarded linen, mattresses, beddings contaminated with blood or body fluid	Nonchlorinated yellow plastic bags or suitable packing material	Nonchlorinated chemical disinfection followed by incineration or plasma Pyrolysis or for energy recovery. In absence of above facilities, shredding or mutilation or combination of sterilization and shredding. Treated waste to be sent for energy recovery or incineration or plasma pyrolysis
	h. **Microbiology, biotechnology, and other clinical laboratory waste:** Blood bags, laboratory cultures, stocks, or specimens of microorganisms, live or attenuated vaccines, human and animal cell cultures used in research, industrial laboratories, production of biological, residual toxins, dishes, and devices used for cultures	Autoclave safe plastic bags or containers	Pretreat to sterilize with nonchlorinated chemicals on-site as per National AIDS Control Organization or World Health Organization guidelines thereafter for incineration
Red	**Contaminated waste (recyclable):** Wastes generated from disposable items, such as tubing, bottles, intravenous tubes and sets, catheters, urine bags, syringes (without needles and fixed needle syringes) and vacutainers (with their needles cut) and gloves	Red-colored nonchlorinated plastic bags or containers	Autoclaving or microwaving/hydroclaving followed by shredding or mutilation or combination of sterilization and shredding. Treated waste to be sent to registered or authorized recyclers or for energy recovery or plastics to diesel or fuel oil or for road making, whichever is possible. Plastic waste should not be sent to landfill sites.

Contd...

Contd...

Category	Type of waste	Types of bag or container to be used	Treatment and disposal options
(1)	(2)	(3)	(4)
White (translu-cent)	**Waste sharps including metals:** Needles, syringes with fixed needles, needles from needle tip cutter or burner, scalpels, blades, or any other contaminated sharp object that may cause puncture and cuts. This includes both used, discarded, and contaminated metal sharps	Puncture proof, leak proof, tamper proof containers	Autoclaving or dry heat sterilization followed by shredding or mutilation or encapsulation in metal container or cement concrete; combination of shredding cum autoclaving; and sent for final disposal to iron foundries (having consent to operate from the State Pollution Control Boards or Pollution Control Committees) or sanitary landfill or designated concrete waste sharp pit
Blue	a. **Glassware:** Broken or discarded and contaminated glass including medicine vials and ampoules except those contaminated with cytotoxic wastes	Cardboard boxes with blue-colored marking	Disinfection (by soaking the washed glass waste after cleaning with detergent and sodium hypochlorite treatment) or through autoclaving or microwaving or hydroclaving and then sent for recycling
	b. **Metallic body implants**	Cardboard boxes with blue-colored marking	
	Part-II		

1. All plastic bags shall be as per BIS standards as and when published, till then the prevailing Plastic Waste Management Rules shall be applicable.
2. Chemical treatment using at least 10% sodium hypochlorite having 30% residual chlorine for 20 minutes any other equivalent chemical reagent that should demonstrate efficiency for microorganisms as given in Schedule-III.
3. Mutilation or shredding must be to an extent to prevent unauthorized reuse.

Contd...

Contd...

4. There will be no chemical pretreatment before incineration, except for microbiological, laboratory, and highly infectious waste.
5. Incineration ash (ash from incineration of any biomedical waste) shall be disposed through hazardous waste treatment, storage, and disposal facility (TSDF), if toxic or hazardous constituents are present beyond the prescribed limits as given in the Hazardous Waste (Management, Handling, and Transboundary Movement) Rules, 2008 or as revised from time to time.
6. Dead fetus below the viability period (as per the Medical Termination of Pregnancy Act 1971, amended from time to time) can be considered as human anatomical waste. Such waste should be handed over to the operator of common biomedical waste treatment and disposal facility in yellow bag with a copy of the official Medical Termination of Pregnancy certificate from the Obstetrician or the Medical Superintendent of hospital or healthcare establishment.
7. Cytotoxic drug vials shall not be handed over to unauthorized person under any circumstances. These shall be sent back to the manufactures for necessary disposal at a single point. As a second option, these may be sent for incineration at common bio-medical waste treatment and disposal facility or TSDFs or plasma pyrolysis is at temperature >1,200°C.
8. Residual or discarded chemical wastes, used or discarded disinfectants and chemical sludge can be disposed at hazardous waste TSDF. In such case, the waste should be sent to hazardous waste TSDF through operator of common biomedical waste treatment and disposal facility only.
9. On-site pretreatment of laboratory waste, microbiological waste, blood samples, and blood bags should be disinfected or sterilized as per the Guidelines of World Health Organization or National AIDS Control Organization and then given to the common biomedical waste treatment and disposal facility.
10. Installation of in-house incinerator is not allowed. However, in case there is no common biomedical facility nearby, the same may be installed by the occupier after taking authorization from the State Pollution Control Board.
11. Syringes should be either mutilated or needles should be cut and or stored in tamper proof, leak proof and puncture proof containers for sharps storage. Wherever the occupier is not linked to a disposal facility it shall be theresponsibility of the occupier to sterilize and dispose in the manner prescribed.
12. Biomedical waste generated in households during healthcare activities shall be segregated as per these rules and handed over in separate bags or containers to municipal waste collectors. Urban local bodies shall have tie up withthe common bio-medical waste treatment and disposal facility to pickup this waste from the Material Recovery Facility (MRF) or from the house hold directly, for final disposal in the manner as prescribed in this Schedule.

*Disposal by deep burial is permitted only in rural or remote areas where there is no access to common BMW treatment facility. This will be carried out with prior approval from the prescribed authority and as per the Standards specified in Schedule-III. The deep burial facility shall be located as per the provisions and guidelines issued by Central Pollution Control Board from time totime.

The chimneys of incinerators should be 30 m high and combustion efficiency (CE) of the incinerator should be at least 99%.

Advantage of Incinerator

The incinerator has an advantage of dealing with all pathological and cytotoxic wastes. Body parts, animal waste, microbiological waste, and soiled dressings can be treated with this technique.

Disadvantages of Incinerator

1. It generates highly toxic gases [e.g., dioxins and furans, if polyvinyl chloride (PVC) plastics are present].
2. It adversely affects the health of the community.
3. Recycling and reprocessing of materials cannot be done.
4. Burning of plastic waste or sharps is also not recommended.

2. Chemical Disinfection

Chemicals are added to waste to kill or inactivate the pathogens it contains. This is a very useful method for many items, particularly in small places. Chemical disinfection is most suitable for treating liquid waste, such as blood, urine, stools or hospital sewage. However, solid wastes including microbiological cultures, sharps, etc., may also be disinfected chemically with certain limitations.

3. Wet and Dry Thermal Treatment

Wet Thermal Treatment

Wet thermal treatment or steam disinfection is based on exposure of shredded infectious waste to high temperature, high pressure steam, and is similar to the autoclave sterilization process. The process is inappropriate for the treatment of anatomical waste and animal carcasses, and will not efficiently treat chemical and pharmaceutical waste.

Screw-feed Technology

Screw-feed technology is the basis of a nonburn, dry, and thermal disinfection process in which waste is shredded and heated in a rotating auger. The waste is reduced by 80% in volume and by 20–35% in weight. This process is suitable for treating infectious waste and sharps, but it should not be used to process pathological, cytotoxic, or radioactive waste.

4. Microwave Irradiation

This is another useful method of sterilization of small volume waste at the point of generation. Most microorganisms are destroyed by the action of microwave of a frequency of about 2,450 MHz and a wavelength of 12.24 cm. The water contained within the waste is rapidly heated by the microwaves and the infectious components are destroyed by heat conduction. This cannot be used for animal or human body parts, metal items, or toxic or radioactive material.

The efficiency of the microwave disinfection should be checked routinely through bacteriological and virological tests.

5. Land Disposal

If a municipality or medical authority genuinely lacks the means to treat waste before disposal, the use of a landfill has to be regarded as an acceptable disposal route. There are two types of disposal land- **open dumps** and **sanitary landfills**. Healthcare waste should not be deposited on or around open dumps. The risk of either people or animals coming into contact with infectious pathogens is obvious.

6. Inertization

The process of "inertization" involves mixing waste with cement and other substances before disposal, in order to minimize the risk of toxic substances contained in the wastes migrating into the surface water or ground water. A typical proportion of the mixture is—65% pharmaceutical waste, 15% lime, 15% cement, and 5% water. A homogeneous mass is formed and cubes or pellets are produced on site and then transported to suitable storage sites.

■ BIOMEDICAL WASTE MANAGEMENT IN INDIA

National legislation is the basis for improving healthcare waste disposal practices in any country. It establishes legal control, and permits the national agency responsible for the disposal of healthcare waste, usually the Ministry of Health, to apply pressure for their implementation. The Ministry of Environment may also be involved. There should be a clear designation of responsibilities before the law is enacted.

The United Nations Conference on the Environment and Development (UNCED) in 1992 recommended the following measures:
a. Prevent and minimize waste production
b. Reuse or recycle the waste to the extent possible
c. Treat waste by safe and environmentally sound methods, and
d. Dispose off the final residue by landfill in confined and carefully designed sites

Biomedical waste (Management and Handling) Rule 1998, prescribed by the Ministry of Environment and Forests, Government of India, came into force on 28th July 1998. This rule applies to those who generate, collect, receive, store, dispose, treat or handle BMW in any manner. **Table 17.1** shows the categories of BMW, types of waste, and treatment and disposal options under rule 1998. The Act is superseded by Biomedical Waste Management rules 2016. **Table 17.1** shows the categories of BMW, types of waste, and treatment and disposal options under rule 2016. The 2016 rules have been amended in 2018 and 2019.

The BMW should be segregated into containers bags at the point of generation of the waste. The color coding and the type of containers used for disposal of waste are as shown in **Table 17.1**.

Waste Management Program

All laboratories should develop waste management program according to the specific needs of the individual laboratory. The policies and procedures should be incorporated in the laboratory's operating manuals. Emphasis should be on waste minimization (by reducing waste, reuse, and recycling), proper segregation, and health and safety of the workers. All personnel generating, collecting, transporting, and storing infectious waste must be trained under the program.

Biosafety

Biosafety can be defined as a group of practices and procedures designed to provide safe environment for individuals who work with

potentially hazardous biological materials in laboratory environments. The primary goal of biosafety to reduce or eliminate exposures to these agents through the use of containment:
- Safety organization
- Safety codes
- Hazards groups
- Containment level

Biomedical Waste Handlers

- Immunize all HCWs and others, involved in handling of BMW for protection against diseases including hepatitis B and tetanus, which are likely to be transmitted by handling of BMW, in a manner as prescribed in the National Immunization Policy or the guidelines of the Ministry of Health and Family Welfare issued from time to time.
- Ensure occupational safety of all HCWs and others involved in handling of BMW by providing appropriate and adequate personal protective equipment (PPE).
- Conduct health check-up at the time of induction and at least once in a year for all HCWs and others involved in handling of BMW and maintain the records for the same.

■ LAUNDRY MANAGEMENT PROCESS

Laundry in a healthcare facility may include bedsheets and blankets, towels, personal clothing, patient apparel, uniforms, scrub suits, gowns, and drapes for surgical procedures. Although, contaminated textiles and fabrics in healthcare facilities can be a source of substantial numbers of pathogenic microorganisms, reports of healthcare-associated diseases linked to contaminated fabrics are so few in number that the overall risk of disease transmission during the laundry process likely is negligible. When the incidence of such events are evaluated in the context of the volume of items laundered in healthcare settings, existing control measures (e.g., standard precautions) are effective in reducing the risk of disease transmission to patients and staff. Therefore, use of current control measures should be continued to minimize the contribution of contaminated laundry to the incidence of healthcare-associated infections.

Chapter 17: Biomedical Waste Management

The **control measures** of the guideline are based on principles of hygiene, common sense, and consensus guidance; they pertain to laundry services utilized by healthcare facilities, either in-house or contract, rather than to laundry done in the home. The purpose of the laundry portion of the standard is to protect the worker from exposure to potentially infectious materials during collection, handling, and sorting of contaminated textiles through the use of personal protective equipment, proper work practices, containment, labeling, hazard communication, and ergonomics. Laundry facility is usually partitioned into two separate areas—a **"dirty" area** for receiving and handling the soiled laundry and **a "clean" area** for processing the washed items. To minimize the potential for recontaminating cleaned laundry with aerosolized contaminated lint, areas receiving contaminated textiles should be at negative air pressure relative to the clean areas. Laundry areas should have hand-washing facilities readily available to workers. Laundry workers should wear appropriate personal protective equipment (e.g., gloves and protective garments) while sorting soiled fabrics and textiles. Laundry equipment should be used and maintained according to the manufacturer's instructions to prevent microbial contamination of the system. Damp textiles should not be left in machines overnight.

KEY POINTS

- **Biomedical waste (BMW)** means any waste, which is generated during the diagnosis, treatment, or immunization of human beings or animals or in research activities pertaining thereto or in the production or testing of biologicals.
- **Waste segregation:** Waste should be segregated in bags of different colors to facilitate appropriate treatment and disposal.
- There are various techniques of biomedical wastes. These include incineration, autoclaving, microwaving, hydroclaving, plasma torch, and chemical treatment.

IMPORTANT QUESTIONS

1. Describe various techniques used for the treatment and disposal of hospital waste.
2. Write short notes on:
   a. Segregation of waste
   b. Hospital waste management of biomedical waste

MULTIPLE CHOICE QUESTIONS (MCQs)

1. Categories of waste for contaminated plastic waste is:
   a. Yellow
   b. Red
   c. White translucent
   d. Blue
2. All is true about incineration, *except*:
   a. It is a high temperature dry oxidation process.
   b. This is a safe method of treating large solid infectious waste.
   c. The incinerator subjects them to very high heat, converting them to ash.
   d. It is cheap and is generally used only by very large establishments.
3. Chemical disinfection is recommended for treatment of:
   a. Laboratory glassware
   b. Liquid waste, such as blood, urine, stools or hospital sewage
   c. Laundry in a healthcare facility
   d. For distinction of gloves

ANSWERS
1. b   2. d   3. b

SECTION 6
Introduction to Laboratory Techniques

Section Outline

- ❖ Microscopy
- ❖ Staining Methods
- ❖ Identification of Common Microbes under the Microscope

CHAPTER 18

Microscopy

Learning Objectives

After reading and studying this chapter, you should be able to:
- Discuss microscopic methods.
- Explain the parts of a microscope.
- Describe the care of microscope.

■ INTRODUCTION

Microscope is an optical instrument used to magnify (enlarge) minute objects or microorganisms which cannot be seen by naked eye. The study of the morphology of bacteria requires the use of microscopes. In general, microscopy is used in microbiology for two basic purposes: (1) the **initial detection of microbes** and (2) **the preliminary or definitive identification of microbes**.

■ MICROSCOPY: INSTRUMENTS

Microscopic Methods

A. **Light Microscopy**
   1. Bright-field (light) microscope
   2. Dark-field microscopy
   3. Phase-contrast microscopy
   4. Fluorescent microscopy
   5. Confocal microscopy
B. **Electron Microscopy**
   1. Transmission
   2. Scanning
C. **Scanning Probe Microscopes**

Light Microscopy

Light microscopy refers to the use of any kind of microscope that uses visible light to observe specimens. Here we examine several types of light microscopy. A modern **compound light microscope (LM)** has a series of lenses and uses visible light as its source of illumination (**Fig. 18.1**).

Principles of Light Microscopy: The Bright-field Microscope

In light microscopy, light typically passes through a specimen and then through a series of magnifying lenses. The most common type of light microscope, and the easiest to use, is the **bright-field microscope**, which evenly illuminates the field of view.

Compound Light Microscopy

A. Parts of Microscope

The following is a description of the parts and function of a compound microscope (**Fig. 18.1**). An ordinary light microscope consists of different parts such as the stand, the optical system, the body, the stage, the substage and the mirror (**Fig. 18.1**).

1. **Stand:** The upright *stand* rests on a heavy *foot* and bears at its upper end an inclined binocular head with two *eye-pieces* (1), above, and a revolving *nose-piece* (3) bearing several *objectives*, below. The stand rests on a heavy *foot* and the *limb* which bears the optical system.

2. **The optical system:** The stand bears at its upper end an inclined binocular head with two *eye-pieces*, above with (magnification 5X, 6X or 10X), and a revolving *nose-piece* bearing several *objectives*, below with different focal lengths and thus different magnifying powers. The three objectives most commonly used in microbiology are: (1) a low-power "dry" objective with focal length 16 mm and magnification x 10, (2) a high-power "dry" objective with focal length 4 mm and magnification x 40, and (3) an oil-immersion objective with focal length "2 mm" and magnification x 100. The 100X objective must only be used with a drop of immersion oil between it and the slide.

   Magnification: We can calculate the **total magnification** of a specimen by multiplying the objective lens magnification (power)

Chapter 18: Microscopy 197

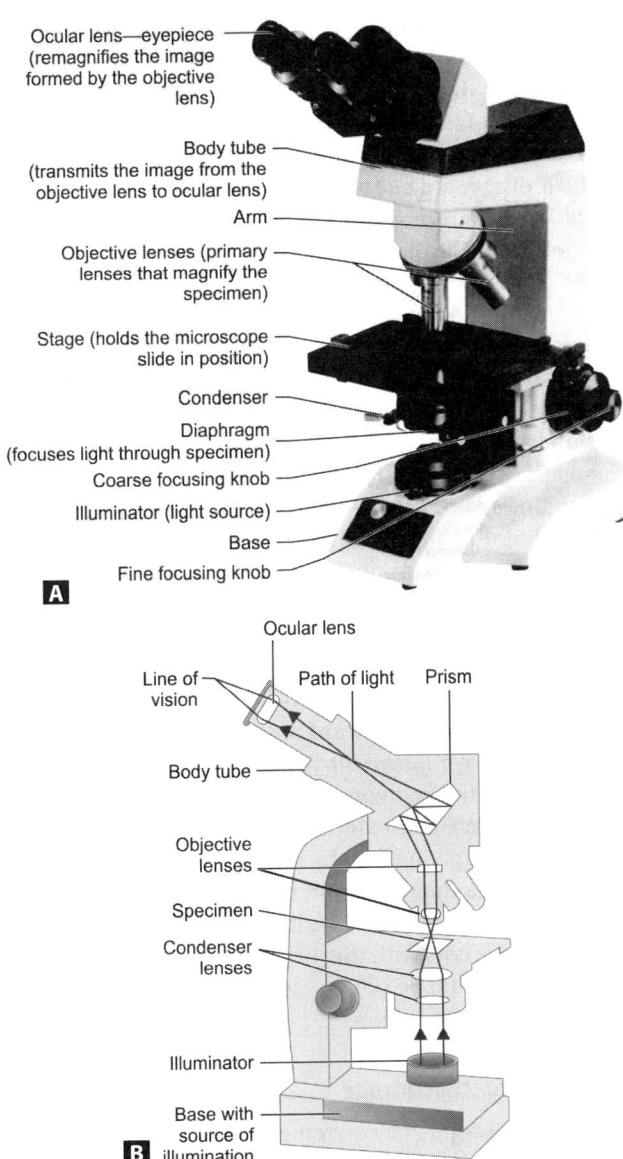

Figs. 18.1A and B: The compound light microscope: (A) Principal parts and functions; (B) The path of light (bottom to top).

by the ocular lens magnification (power). Three different objective lenses are commonly used—(1) **low power (10X); (2) high dry (40X); and (3) oil immersion (100X)**. Most oculars magnify specimens by a factor of 10. Multiplying the magnification of a specific objective lens with that of the ocular, we see that the total magnifications would be 100X for low power, 400X for high power, and 1000X for oil immersion.

3. **The stage:** This is the platform on which material (i.e., the "object") is placed to be examined.
   Attached through a racking mechanism to the middle of the stand is a horizontal platform, or *stage,* with a central hole over which the slide with specimen is held by clips. The specimen can be centered with the "mechanical stage adjustment knob", so that object can be moved from side to side and before backward.
   For focusing, the stage is racked upward or downward by turning the milled heads of *coarse* and *fine focusing adjustments*. For searching different areas of the specimen, the slide can be moved in two directions by turning *mechanical stage adjustments*.

4. **The substage:** A built-in *lamp* in the foot of the microscope passes a beam of light upward through a *field diaphragm* (iris). The beam is focused on to the specimen by a *substage condenser* which is attached beneath the stage, centered by condenser centration adjustments and moved upward or downward by the turning of a *condenser focusing adjustment.* An *aperture diaphragm* (iris) with a lever for its control is incorporated in the condenser mounting.
   Magnification: We can calculate the **total magnification** of a specimen by multiplying the objective lens magnification (power) by the ocular lens magnification (power). Most oculars magnify specimens by a factor of 10. Multiplying the magnification of a specific objective lens with that of the ocular, we see that the total magnifications would be 100X for low power, 400X for high power, and 1000X for oil immersion.

Methods of Use of Light Microscope

1. Place the microscope at a convenient position on the bench and adjust the height and position of the observer's chair, so that prolonged viewing may be done in comfort.
2. Check to ensure that the objectives and eye-pieces are free from dust and immersion oil.

3. Rack up fully the substage condenser, i.e., until its top surface is within about 1 mm below the upper surface of the stage (undersurface of the slide).
4. Check that the filter carrier in the substage is in its correct position and not in an intermediate position where it will obscure the light.
5. Fully open the substage and lamp irises.
6. Switch on the lamp at low intensity and then increase the intensity.
7. Place the slide with the object on the stage, so that it is held by the stage clips and pressed at both ends into close contact with the surface of the stage.
8. First view the specimen with a low power dry objective and use the coarse focusing adjustment to focus the specimen on the slide. Move an area of the slide with easily visible material into the centre of the field, where it will be available in the smaller field to be focused with the high-power objectives.

    Note: Never use the fine focusing adjustment until the specimen has been made visible and brought nearly into focus with the coarse adjustment. Use the fine adjustment only to obtain and maintain exact focus.

9. Adjust the distance between the eye-pieces so that a single field is seen.
10. If continued examination with the **low power objective** is required, diffuse the light uniformly over the field by defocusing the condenser either by racking it down or swinging out its top lens. Reduce the illumination by turning down the intensity control of the lamp, not by closing the iris diaphragm of the substage or lamp.
11. Before proceeding to use a **high-power objective**, check that the iris diaphragms are open, the condenser is focused by fully racking up and that the illumination is properly centered.
12. Before using an **oil-immersion objective**, rack down the stage to give adequate clearance between the slide and the objective, and place a moderately large drop of immersion oil on the middle of the specimen central to the light beam focused from the condenser. Take care not to spill oil on the microscope.

    i. Rotate the nose-piece until the oil immersion lens is in position.

    ii. With the eye at the level of the stage, use the *coarse* focusing adjustment slowly to raise the stage until the oil on the slide makes contact with the objective and the oil "lights up". Then, still with the coarse adjustment, raise the stage a little further to bring the surface of the slide as close as possible to the objective lens without actually touching it. Take care to avoid damaging the lens by pressing it against the slide.

13. Apply the eyes to the eye-pieces and, while watching, slowly focus the objective *away* from the slide by lowering the stage with the coarse focusing adjustment. Stop as soon as focus is reached and the specimen is seen. Then, and only then, obtain and maintain exact focus by use of the fine adjustment.
14. If focus is missed, do *not* focus back again while looking into the eye-pieces, for the slide might then accidentally be brought into contact with the objective lens.
15. If the illumination is poor, check that it is properly centered before turning up the intensity control on the lamp.
16. Search the specimen in an orderly way by moving the adjustments of the mechanical stage. Keep a hand on the fine focusing adjustment in order to maintain exact focus during the movements of the slide.
17. Wipe the oil from the objective with a clean tissue after use, and clean off any oil that has been spilt on the stage or elsewhere, on the microscope. Turn down the light intensity control to low and then switch off the light.

■ CARE OF THE MICROSCOPE

1. It should be kept at a uniform temperature and not exposed to sunlight or any source of heat.
2. The microscope is a delicate and expensive instrument. It should be moved with care to avoid jarring and mechanical damage, and should be lifted by its fixed upright and foot, not by any moveable part.
3. It should be protected from dust in its box or under a plastic cover when not in use.
4. It should be cleaned at intervals and its working surfaces should be very lightly smeared with soft paraffin. The component parts of objectives or condensers must not be unscrewed or dismantled for cleaning.
5. The lenses of the ocular, objectives, and condenser should be cleaned before and after using the microscope.

6. *Oil-immersion lens should be cleaned after use each day* by wiping with a well-washed, fine cotton cloth (handkerchief or, preferably, with the fine paper tissue). A soiled cloth or tissue must not be used, as it may bear grit that will scratch the lens.
7. Oil left on a lens for a day or more dries becomes sticky and finally hardens, so that it cannot be removed by simple wiping. It should be removed by repeated wiping with a cloth or tissue soaked in benzol or xylol. Alcohol, acetone, chloroform and other solvents must *not* be used, as they may dissolve the cement holding the lenses and so spoil the objective.
8. Eye-pieces from time to time may become contaminated internally with dust, so that fuzzy check specks are seen in the field. When the position of the dirt has been located, remove it with a soft camel-hair brush that has been held for a few seconds against a hot electric bulb. If this fails, use a lens paper moistened with *distilled* water. Dust may collect on the prisms in the binocular head in binocular microscopes. It may be cleaned away with a soft camel-hair brush passed down the eye-piece tubes after removal of the eye-pieces.

KEY POINTS

Microscopy

- In light microscopy, visible light passes through the specimen.
- A simple microscope consists of one lens; a compound microscope has multiple lenses.

Compound Light Microscope

- The most common microscope used in microbiology is the compound microscope/bright-field microscope/light microscope.
- The compound light microscope uses visible light.
- The usefulness of a microscope depends on its resolving power.

IMPORTANT QUESTION

1. Name various microscopic instruments used in microbiology and describe the working principle of compound microscope.

MULTIPLE CHOICE QUESTIONS (MCQs)

1. Which of the following is not a modification of a compound microscope?
   a. Bright microscopy
   b. Dark-field microscopy
   c. Electron microscopy
   d. Phase contrast microscopy
2. Which objective lenses are commonly used?
   a. Low power
   b. High dry
   c. Oil immersion
   d. All of the above

ANSWERS

1. b   2. d

Staining Methods

Learning Objectives

After reading and studying this chapter, you should be able to:
- Describe common staining techniques.
- Describe the following: Simple stains; differential stains; Gram stain; acidfast stain (Ziehl-Neelsen staining of acid-fast bacilli); Albert's stain.

■ INTRODUCTION

The morphological features of an organism can be studied by examining them under using unstained and stained preparations.

Examination of Living Bacteria in Unstained Preparations

The unstained preparations of living organisms can be studied by anyone of the following methods:
1. Wet coverslip preparation
2. Hanging drop preparation
3. Phase contrast microscope
4. Dark ground microscope

Wet Coverslip Preparation

"Wet" mounts, i.e., unstained preparations of fluid material, are widely used in looking at cells in urine, cerebrospinal fluid (CSF), feces, and vaginal secretions. They are ideal rapid methods (takes more than 5 or 10 minutes).

Hanging Drop Preparation

It is done to demonstrate motility and to study morphology of bacteria **(Fig. 19.1)**.
- **Motility:** Motile or non-motile
- **Morphology:** Cocci, bacilli, or coccobacilli

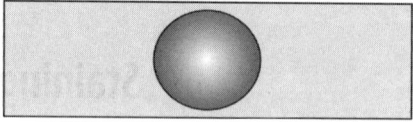

Step 1 – Glass slide containing a plasticin ring

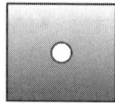

Step 2 – Coverslip with a drop of culture medium

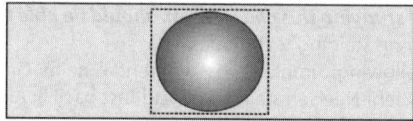

Step 3 – Inverted glass slide from step 1 placed on to overslip in step 2

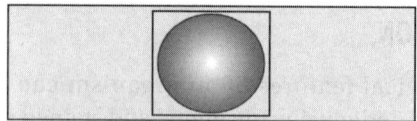

Step 4 – Glass slide in step 3 is turned upside down

Fig. 19.1: Hanging drop preparation.

Requirements
1. A clean cavity (depression) slide
2. A clean coverslip
3. Young broth culture
4. Wire loop
5. Bunsen burner/spirit lamp
6. Microscope

Procedure
1. A "hollow ground" slide (a glass slide with a shallow, circular concavity in its center) is used for *hanging drop preparation.*
2. Encircle the concavity with a line streak of soft petroleum jelly applied with a glass rod to the surface of the slide just outside the concavity.
3. Place drop of culture using the sterile wire loop on the center of the coverslip.

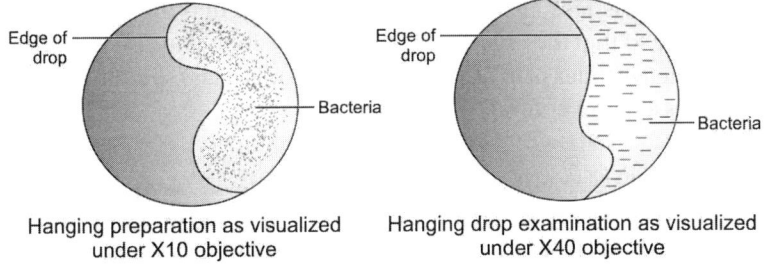

Fig. 19.2: Examination of hanging drop preparation under the microscope.

4. Invert the cavity slide over the coverslip so that the drop of the culture is in the center of the cavity; press it lightly, so that the coverslip adheres to the Vaseline ring.
5. Then quickly turn round the slide, so that the coverslip is uppermost. The drop will then be hanging from the coverslip in the center of the concavity, that is why it is called *hanging drop*.
6. Proceed to examine first with a **low-power objective** and then with a **high-power one**.
7. First focus the edge of a hanging drop preparation under **low-power objective (X10)** of microscope, after reducing the light intensity (by partial closing of iris diaphragm) so that the edge of the drop is exactly in the center of the microscopic field.
8. Turn high-power objective (X40) into position and focus the edge of the hanging drop and observe for the motility and morphology of bacteria. Their shape, approximate size, and general structure can be observed **(Fig. 19.2)**.

Note: Instead of slide with a shallow, circular concavity, in many institutions, plasticine is provided to students. Make a ring of plasticine and place it in the center of a clean glass slide. Invert the glass slide containing the plasticine ring and place it on the coverslip. Rest procedure is the same.

Reasons for Focusing the Edge of the Drop

The edge of the drop is focused to observe the motility and morphology for the following reasons:
- The concentration of the organism is more at the edge because:
  - Aerobic organisms tend to move toward the edge.
  - Surface tension is less at the edge; hence the concentration of organisms is more.

❖ Density is less at the edge of the drop; hence the contrast is better so that the organisms are clearly visible. The differences in refractive index of light rays that pass through glass slide and liquid gives a better contrast at the edge.

Important Points for Observing Motility of Organisms

When examining living organisms for the property of active locomotion, it is essential to distinguish **true motility**, whereby the organisms move in different directions and change their positions in the field, from either:
1. **Passive drifting** of the organisms in the same direction in a convectional current in the fluid or
2. **Brownian movement**, which is an oscillatory movement about a nearly fixed point possessed by all small bodies suspended in fluid and due to irregularities in their bombardment by molecules of water.

Motile Gram-negative Bacilli

- *Escherichia coli*
- *Proteus*
- *Salmonella* sp.
- *Enterobacter*
- *Citrobacter*
- *Hafnia*
- *Serratia* sp.
- *Morganella morganii*
- *Providencia stuartii, rettgeri*
- *Chromobacterium violaceum*
- *Pseudomonas aeruginosa*
- *Burkholderia cepacia*
- *Burkholderia pseudomallei*
- *Vibrio cholerae*
- *Campylobacter*
- *Helicobacter*
- *Clostridium tetani*

Non-motile Gram-negative Bacteria

- *Klebsiella pneumoniae*
- *Shigella* spp.

- *Burkholderia mallei*
- *Streptococcus moniliformis*
- *Gardnerella vaginalis*
- *Flavobacterium menigosepticum*
- Anaerobes:
    - *Bacteroides fragilis*
    - *Fusobacterium* sp.
    - *Leptotrichia buccalis*
    - *Prevotella* spp.
    - *Porphyromonas* sp.

■ METHODS OF STAINING

Because most microorganisms appear almost colorless when viewed through a standard light microscope, we often must prepare them for observation. Live bacteria do not show much structural detail under the light microscope due to lack of contrast. Hence, it is customary to use staining techniques to produce color contrast.

Preparing Film or Smear for Staining

Slides

Film preparations are made either on coverslips or on 3 × 1 in glass slides, usually the latter. It is essential that the coverslips or slides be perfectly clean and free from grease.

Smear preparation: A thin film of material containing the microorganisms is spread over the surface of the slide. This film, called a **smear**, is allowed to air dry.

Fixation: Before the microorganisms can be stained, however, they must be fixed (attached) to the microscope slide. In most staining procedures the slide is fixed by passing it through the flame of a Bunsen burner several times, smear side up. Air drying and flaming fix the microorganisms to the slide. Fixing simultaneously kills the microorganisms and attaches them to the slide. It also preserves various parts of microbes in their natural state with only minimal distortion.

Staining: Stain is applied and then washed off with water; then the slide is blotted with absorbent paper. Without fixing, the stain might wash the microbes off the slide. The stained microorganisms are now ready for microscopic examination.

Types of Stain

Basic dyes: Dyes, which include crystal violet, methylene blue, malachite green, and safranin are more commonly used than acidic dyes.
Acidic dyes: These are eosin, acid fuchsin, and nigrosin.

Negative staining: Preparing colorless bacteria against a colored background is called **negative staining**. It is valuable in the observation of overall cell shapes, sizes, and capsules.

Stained Preparations

Staining simply means coloring the micro-organisms with a dye that emphasizes certain structures. Routine methods for staining of bacteria involve drying and fixing smears, procedures.

■ COMMON STAINING TECHNIQUES

- ❖ Simple stains
- ❖ Differential stains
  - Gram stain
  - Acid-fast stain [Ziehl-Neelsen staining of acid-fast bacilli (AFB)]
- ❖ Special stains
  - Negative staining
  - Impregnation methods:

Simple Stains

Some of the simple stains commonly used in the laboratory are **methylene blue, carbol fuchsin, crystal violet, and safranin.**

Differential Stains

Gram stain and the **acid-fast stain** are two most widely used differential stains.

Gram Stain

It was first devised by the histologist Hans Christian Gram (1884) as a method of staining bacteria in tissues. It is one of the most useful staining procedures because it classifies bacteria into two large groups—Gram-positive and Gram-negative.

Reagents

- **Violet dye:** Crystal violet or methyl violet is used at concentrations of 0.5-2%. Solution is facilitated, if the dye is first dissolved in alcohol and then added to the water.
  - Crystal violet or methyl violet 6B—10 g
  - Absolute alcohol (100% ethanol)—100 mL
  - Distilled water—1 L
- **Gram's iodine:**
  - Iodine—10 g
  - Potassium iodide—20 g
  - Distilled water—1 L
- **Decolorizer:**
  - Acetone
  - Absolute alcohol (100% ethanol)
  - Acetone-alcohol: This is a mixture of 1 volume of acetone with 1 volume of 95% ethanol. It requires application for about 10 seconds.
- **Safranin counterstain:** Safranin 0.5% in distilled water.

Procedure

1. Heat-fixed smear is covered with a basic purple dye, usually **crystal violet (primary stain)** for **1 minute**.
2. Wash the smear thoroughly with water.
3. Cover the smear with Gram's iodine for **1 minute**.
4. Wash again with water.
5. Decolorize the smear with acetone for **10 seconds or less** taking care not to over decolorize (alcohol can be substituted for acetone).
6. Immediately wash with water to remove the decolorizer.
7. Cover the slide with dye safranin (counterstain) for **1 minute**.
8. Wash off the smear with water, blot and dry.
9. Examine the stained smear under the 100 X (oil) immersion objective of the microscope (**Fig. 19.1**).

Interpretation of Gram Stain (Fig. 19.3 and Table 19.1)

Two broad groups:
1. **Gram-positive:** Gram-positive bacteria are those that resist decolorization and retain the primary stain, appearing violet.

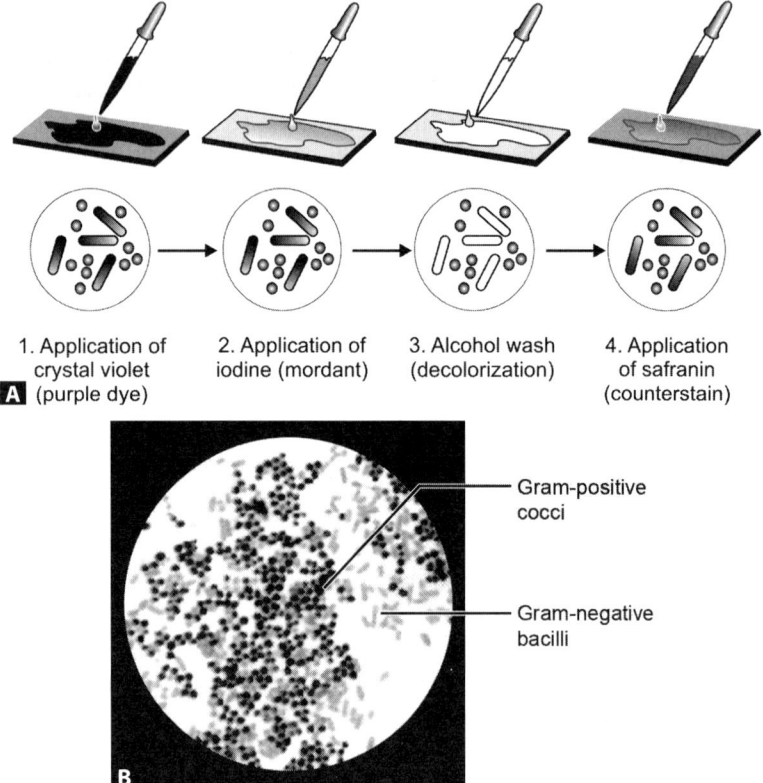

Figs. 19.3A and B: Gram stain: (A) Steps in the Gram stain procedure; (B) Results of a Gram stain. The Gram-positive cells (purple) are *Staphylococcus aureus*; the Gram-negative cells (reddish-pink) are *Escherichia coli*. *(For color version see Plate 1)*

2. **Gram-negative:** Gram-negative bacteria are decolorized by organic solvents (acetone/alcohol) and, therefore, take the counterstain, appearing red.

Gram Staining Mechanism

The exact mechanism is not understood. It may, however, be attributed to following:

1. **Protoplasm:** There is more **acidic protoplasm in the Gram-positive cells,** which is responsible for retaining the basic dye more strongly than the Gram-negative bacteria.

TABLE 19.1: Gram-positive and negative bacteria.

Gram-positive bacteria	Gram-negative bacteria
Cocci ❖ Staphylococcus ❖ Streptococcus ❖ Enterococcus Gram-positive diplococci- Streptococcus pneumoniae	Cocci Bacillus Neisseria

Bacilli
❖ Corynebacterium
❖ Bacillus
❖ Clostridium
❖ Lactobacillus
❖ Mycobacterium
(Some, Mycobacteria, including Mycobacterium tuberculosis are stained only faintly or not at all by Gram's method)
- Actinomyces
- Nocardia
	Bacilli
	❖ Enterobacteria
	  - Escherichia coli
	  - Klebsiella
	  - Salmonella
	  - Shigella
	  - Proteus
	  - Yersinia
	❖ Vibrio
	❖ Pseudomonas
	❖ Parvobacteria
	  - Haemophilus
	  - Bordetella
	  - Brucella
	❖ Bacteroides

2. **Cell wall structure:** Different kinds of bacteria react differently to the gram stain, because of structural differences in their cell walls.

   Gram-positive cells: Gram-positive bacteria have a **thicker peptidoglycan cell wall** than Gram-negative bacteria. The complex **crystal violet-iodine (CV-I) complex** is larger than the CV molecule that entered the cells, and, because of its size, it cannot be washed out of the intact peptidoglycan layer of Gram-positive cells by **acetone/alcohol**. Consequently, Gram-positive cells retain the color of the CV dye.

   Gram-negative: Gram-negative bacterial cell walls are **thinner**, have a **smaller amount of peptidoglycan** and contain a high percentage of lipids. There is a layer of lipopolysaccharide as part of their cell wall. They dissolve during treatment with acetone alcohol, forming **larger pores** in the cell wall, and the **CV-I complex** is washed out through the thin layer of peptidoglycan. Causing outflow of dye-iodine complex and take up counter stain, thus appearing red/pink (Gram-negative).

Cell wall integrity: It has been found that Gram-positivity depends on the integrity of cell wall and presence of specific magnesium-ribonucleate-protein complex. The Gram-positive bacteria become Gram-negative when cell wall is damaged.

Acid-Fast Stain (Ziehl-Neelsen Staining of Acid-fast Bacilli)

Acid-fast stain was discovered by Ehrlich (1882), who found that after staining with aniline dyes, tubercle bacilli resist decolorization with acids. The method, as modified by Ziehl and Neelsen, is in common use now.

Principle

Some bacteria such as mycobacteria, are resistant to aniline dyes and do not readily penetrate the substance of the tubercle bacillus and are therefore unsuitable for staining it. The dye can be made to penetrate the bacillus by the use of a powerful staining solution that contains **phenol,** and the **application of heat.** Once stained the tubercle bacillus cannot be decolorized even with powerful decolorizing agents for a considerable time and thus still retains the stain when everything else in the microscopic preparation has been decolorized. Hence, they are called **AFB.**

The stain used consists of **basic fuchsin,** with **phenol** (acts as a mordant) added. The dye is basic and its combination with a mineral acid used as decolorizer produces a compound that is **yellowish-brown in color,** which is readily dissolved out of all structures except acid-fast bacteria. Any strong acid can be used as a decolorizing agent, but 20% sulfuric acid (by volume) is usually employed. In order to show structures and cells, including non-acid-fast bacteria, that have been decolorized, and to form a contrast with the red-stained bacilli, the preparation is counterstained with **methylene blue or malachite green (Fig. 19.4)**.

Acid-fastness has been ascribed to the high content and variety of lipids, fatty acids, and higher alcohols found in tubercle bacilli. A lipid peculiar to AFB, a high-molecular weight hydroxy acid-wax containing carboxyl groups **(mycolic acid)** is acid-fast in the free state. Acid-fastness depends also on the **integrity of the cell wall** besides lipid contents.

Make a smear on a numbered slide, dry and fix by flaming by passing the *dried* slide, film downward, three times slowly through

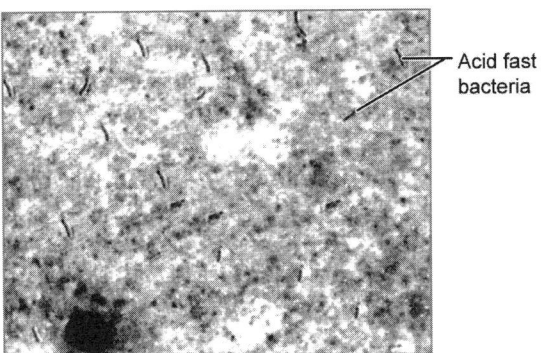

Fig. 19.4: Ziehl-Neelsen stain (100X). *(For color version see Plate 2)*

the flame, or by heating through the glass slide (the slide is held, film upward) in the top of the Bunsen flame for a few seconds so' that the slide becomes hot.

Procedure

1. The slide containing fixed smear is covered with carbol fuchsin. The carbol fuchsin is left on the slide for **5–10 minutes** with intermittent heating during that period. Heat the slide until the steam rises, but without boiling.
   (Do not allow the stain to dry, to counteract drying more solution of stain is added to the slide and the slide reheated).
2. Wash in tap water.
3. The stained smear is decolorized with **20% sulfuric acid.** The red color of the preparation is changed to **yellow brown**. After about 1 minute in the acid, wash the slide with water, and pour on fresh acid. Repeat this procedure several times. When it is complete, the film, after washing, is only very faintly pink.
4. The smear is counterstained with a contrasting dye such as methylene blue for **1–2 minutes**. Malachite green can also be used as counter-stain instead of methylene blue.
5. Wash with water, blot with clean paper, dry, and mount.
6. Examine under oil immersion (X100) objective.

Important Points in Observation

Acid-fast bacilli such as *Mycobacterium tuberculosis* appear red while other organisms, tissue cells, and debris are stained blue or green according to the counterstain used **(Fig. 19.2)**.

Acid-fast Organisms
1. All mycobacteria are acid-fast, e.g., *Mycobacterium tuberculosis, Mycobacterium bovis, Mycobacterium leprae, and* atypical mycobacteria.
2. *Nocardia asteroides, Nocardia brasiliensis*
3. *Cryptosporidium*—a protozoan coccidian parasite, which causes opportunistic infections in AIDS is acid-fast.
4. Bacterial spores are weakly acid-fast.

Ziehl-Neelsen Reagents
1. **Ziehl-Neelsen carbol fuchsin**
   - Basic fuchsin (powder)—5 g
   - Phenol (crystalline)—25 g
   - Alcohol (95% or 100% ethanol)—50 mL
   - Distilled water—500 mL
2. **Sulfuric acid (20%) decolorizer**
   - Concentrated sulfuric acid—250 mL (98%, 1.835 g/mL)
   - Distilled water—1 L
3. **Alcohol 95%:** Ethanol 95 mL plus water to 100 mL, *or* industrial methylated spirit
4. **Acid-alcohol decolorizer**
   - Concentrated hydrochloric acid—75 mL
   - Industrial methylated spirit—2,425 mL
5. **Methylene blue counterstain**
   - Loeffler's methylene blue (see above)
6. **Saturated solution**
   - Methylene blue in alcohol—300 mL
   - KOH, 0.01% in water—1 L

Staining of Volutin Containing Organisms

Well-developed granules of volutin (polyphosphate) may be seen in unstained wet preparations as round refractile bodies within the bacterial cytoplasm. They tend to stain more strongly than the rest of the bacterium with **basic dyes,** and with **toluidine blue or methylene blue** they stain metachromatically, a **reddish-purple color.** They are demonstrated most clearly by special methods, such as Albert's and Neisser's, which stain them dark purple but the remainder of the bacterium with a contrasting counterstain. For routine use the following method is recommended:

Albert's Stain

A fixed smear is provided for Albert's staining. If the smear is unfixed, it is fixed by passing the *dried* slide, film downward, three times slowly through the flame, or by heating through the glass slide (the slide is held, film upward) in the top of the Bunsen flame for a few seconds, so that the slide becomes hot.

Procedure

1. Make film, dry in air, and fix by heat
2. Cover slide with Albert's stain (Albert's solution A) and allow to act for **3–5 minutes**
3. Wash in water and blot dry
4. Cover slide with Albert's iodine (Albert's solution B) for **1 minute**
5. Wash with water and blot dry. Observe under the oil-immersion objective (X100).

The metachromatic (volutin) granules of *Corynebacterium diphtheriae* stain **bluish black**, and the bacterial protoplasm **green** and other organisms mostly **light green (Fig. 19.5)**.

Important Points in Observation

1. In case of *Corynebacterium diphtheriae,* green colored bacilli with bluish black metachromatic (volutin) granules are observed.
2. Bacilli are arranged in *Chinese letter* or *cuneiform arrangement* **(Fig. 19.5)**.

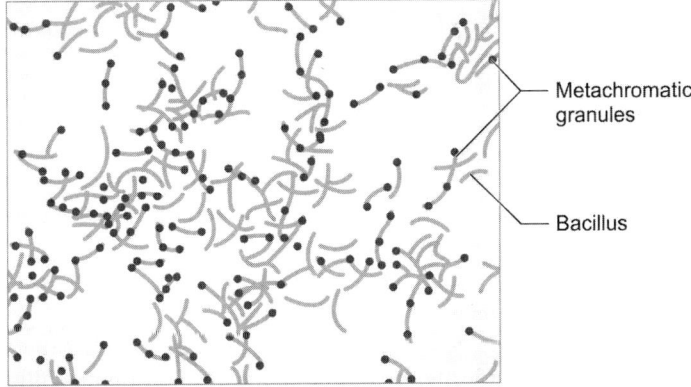

Fig. 19.5: Albert's stain (100X). *(For color version see Plate 2)*

3. Show your observations to the examiner by focusing a good stained field of your smear as such and by drawing a well labeled diagram using colored pencils.

Special Stains

Special stains are used to stain specific structures inside or outside of a cell color and isolate specific parts of microorganisms, such as capsule stain, endospore stain, and flagella stain.

Staining of Capsules

India ink Preparation Procedure

1. Carefully wipe a microscopic slide free from particles of dust or dirt.
2. Place a large loopful of undiluted India ink on the slide.
3. Emulsify a very small portion of solid material culture or a small loopful of liquid culture in the ink.
4. Place a clean coverslip on the ink drop and press it down through a sheet of blotting paper to make the film very thin and thus pale in color.
5. Examine under × **100 to × 1,000 magnification.**
6. The highly refractile outline of the bacterium is seen. Between this refractive surface membrane and the clear background of the particles there is a clear space, which represents the capsule. **The capsule appears as a clear halo around the yeast cell.**

Uses: The India ink method is useful for demonstrating the presence of a capsule **especially *Cryptococcus neoformans*** in clinical specimens, particularly cerebrospinal fluid.

Staining of Spores

- ❖ **Gram stain:** The body of the bacillus is deeply colored, whereas the spore is unstained and appears as a clear halo in the organism.
- ❖ Malachite green stain for spores:
    - Place the slide over a beaker of boiling water, resting it on the rim with the bacterial film uppermost.
    - When, within several seconds, large droplets have condensed on the underside of the slide, flood it with 5% aqueous solution

of malachite green and leave to act for 1 minute while the water continues to boil.
- Wash in cold water.
- Treat with 0.5% safranin or 0.05% basic fuchsin for 30 seconds.
- Wash and dry.
- Examine under oil immersion (X100) objective.
- Spore-colors green; vegetative bacilli-red

■ METHODS FOR DETECTION FOR DIRECT MICROSCOPIC DETECTION OF FUNGI IN CLINICAL SPECIMENS

Potassium Hydroxide (KOH) Preparation

1. A drop of the KOH (10-20%) preparation is added to a slide.
2. An aliquot of specimen (nail scrapings, hair, skin scales, or thin slices of tissue) are added to the drop, and a coverslip is added.
3. The slide is held at room temperature for 5-30 minutes after the addition of KOH, depending on the specimen type, to allow digestion to occur. Digestive capabilities can be enhanced with gentle heating or the addition of 40% dimethyl sulfoxide.
4. Hyaline molds and yeasts appear transparent, while dematiaceous molds may display golden visible brown hyphae. It can be used in combination with calcofluor hydroxide of specimen to make for fluorescence microscopy (KOH) fungi more readily.

Lactophenol Cotton (Aniline) Blue (LPCB) Stain

Needle-mount Method

1. Place a drop of 95% alcohol on the slide. Gently tease out a fragment of the culture in the alcohol with needles or straight wires. When it is satisfactorily spread, let most of the alcohol evaporate and then a drop of stain.
2. Apply a coverslip.
3. Remove any excess stain round the coverslip with the edge of a piece of blotting paper.
4. Examine at X100 to X400 magnification.

Uses: It is commonly used for the microscopic examination of fungal cultures by tease or tape preparation. The addition of 10% polyvinyl alcohol (LPCB-PVA) makes an excellent permanent stain or fixative for mounting slide culture preparations.

KEY POINTS

- Hanging drop preparation: It is done to demonstrate motility and to study morphology of bacteria.
- The Gram stain procedure uses a purple stain (crystal violet), iodine as a mordant, an alcohol decolorizer, and a red counterstain. Gram-positive bacteria stain purple and Gram-negative bacteria stain pink.
- The acid-fast stain is used to stain organisms, such as *Mycobacteria*; acid-fast organisms stain pink and all other organisms stain blue.

IMPORTANT QUESTIONS

1. Describe in detail the Gram's stain. Describe Gram staining mechanism.
2. Give an account of differential stains.
3. Write short notes on:
   a. Simple staining.
   b. Acid-fast stain or Ziehl-Neelsen stain.

MULTIPLE CHOICE QUESTIONS (MCQs)

1. **All include basic dyes, *except*:**
   a. Crystal violet
   b. Methylene blue
   c. Malachite green
   d. Nigrosin
2. **Special stains are used to color and isolate various structures, such as:**
   a. Capsule
   b. Endospore
   c. Flagella
   d. All of the above

ANSWERS

1. d   2. d

CHAPTER 20

Identification of Common Microbes under the Microscope

Learning Objectives

After reading and studying this chapter, you should be able to:
- Explain the role of microscopy in the identification of etiologic agents including bacteria, fungi, viruses, and parasites.
- List the staining methods used to aid in the detection of bacteria in clinical specimens.
- Describe methods for direct detection of fungi, and parasites in clinical specimens.

■ INTRODUCTION

The morphological features of an organism can be studied by examining them under using unstained and stained preparations. The microscopic examination of clinical specimens is used to detect bacterial cells, fungal elements, parasites (eggs, larvae, or adult forms), and viral inclusions present in infected cells. Characteristic morphologic properties can be used for the preliminary identification of most bacteria and are used for the definitive identification of many fungi and parasites. The microscopic detection of organisms stained with antibodies labeled with fluorescent dyes or other markers has proved to be very useful for the specific identification of many organisms.

Wet-mount, heat-fixed, or chemically fixed specimens can be examined with an ordinary bright-field microscope. For bacteriology, the Gram and Ziehl-Neelsen stains are usually sufficient, but for the demonstration of fungi or parasites special stains or concentration techniques may be required.

■ EXAMINATION METHODS

Clinical specimens or suspensions of microorganisms can be placed on a glass slide and examined under the microscope (i.e., direct examination of a wet mount). Although large organisms (e.g., fungal elements, parasites) and cellular material can be seen using this method, analysis of the internal detail is often difficult.

Direct Examination of a Wet Mount

Direct examination methods are the simplest for preparing samples for microscopic examination. **Wet mounts**, i.e., unstained preparations of fluid material, are widely used in looking at cells in urine, cerebrospinal fluid (CSF), feces, and vaginal secretions. They are ideal rapid methods (takes more than 5 or 10 minutes).

Methods for Detection for Direct Microscopic Detection of Bacteria in Clinical Specimens

Staining Methods

1. Gram Stain

The **Gram stain** is the best known and most widely used stain and forms the basis for the phenotypic classification of bacteria. **Yeasts** can also be stained with this method (yeasts are Gram-positive). When clinical material is Gram stained (e.g., the direct smear), the slide is evaluated for the presence of bacterial cells as well as the Gram reactions (**Gram-positive or Gram-negative**), morphologies (e.g., cocci or bacilli), and arrangements (e.g., chains, pairs, clusters) of the cells seen. Similar to direct smears, indirect smears prepared from bacterial growth are evaluated for the bacterial cells' Gram reactions, morphologies, and arrangements (**Fig. 20.1**).

Morphotype Description

Gram-positive Cocci

Examples:
- Chains: *Streptococcus*
- Clusters: *Staphylococcus* spp.
- Gram-positive diplococci (lancet-shaped): *Streptococcus pneumoniae*
- Gram-negative diplococci: Pathogenic *Neisseria* spp.

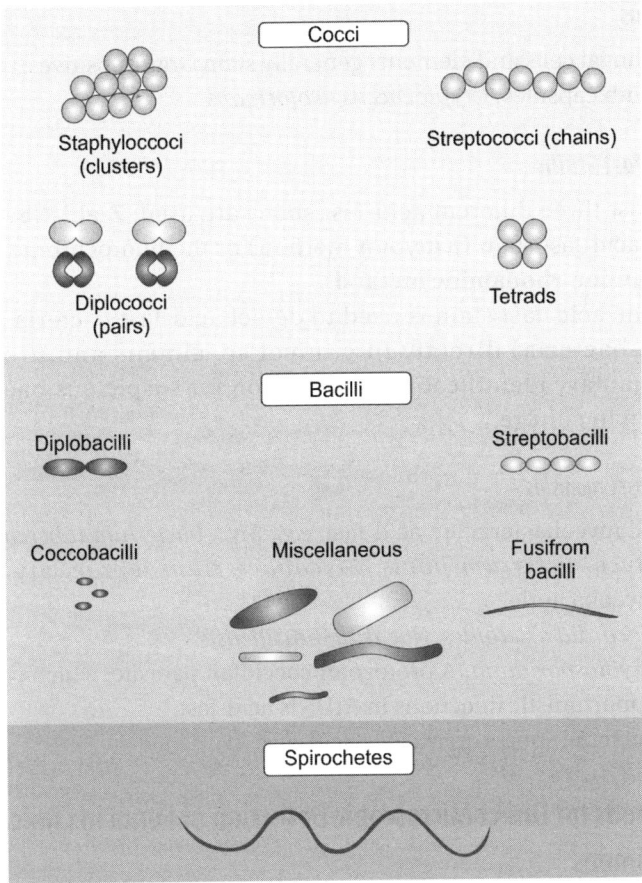

Fig. 20.1: Examples of common bacterial cellular morphologies, Gram staining reactions, and cellular arrangements.

Bacilli

Examples:

Gram-positive bacilli:

- Small: *Listeria monocytogenes, Corynebacterium* spp.

Gram-negative bacilli:

- Gram-negative coccobacilli: *Bordetella, Haemophilus* (pleomorphic)
- Curved: *Vibrio, Campylobacter*

Fungus
- Fungal cells and elements generally stain Gram-positive
- With capsules: *Cryptococcus neoformans*

Acid-fast Stains
At least three different acid-fast stains are used: **Ziehl-Neelsen**, cold acid-fast stain **(Kinyoun method)** or the fluorochrome stain **(auramine-rhodamine method)**.

The acid-fast stain is used to detect acid-fast bacteria (e.g., mycobacteria) directly in clinical specimens and provide preliminary identification information for suspicious bacteria grown in culture.

Acid-fast Organisms
1. All mycobacteria are acid-fast, *e.g., Mycobacterium tuberculosis, Mycobacterium bovis, Mycobacterium leprae,* atypical mycobacteria.
2. *Nocardia asteroides, Nocardia brasiliensis*
3. *Cryptosporidium:* A protozoan coccidian parasite, which causes opportunistic infections in AIDS is acid-fast.
4. Bacterial spores are weakly acid-fast.

Methods for Direct Microscopic Detection of Fungi in Clinical Specimens

Potassium Hydroxide (KOH) Preparation
Potassium hydroxide (KOH) 10% is used to dissolve proteinaceous material and facilitate detection of fungal elements that are not affected by strong alkali solution. It can be used in combination with calcofluor hydroxide of specimen to make for fluorescence microscopy (KOH) fungi more readily.

Lactophenol Cotton Blue (LPCB) Stain
It is commonly used for the microscopic examination of fungal cultures by tease or tape preparation.

Methods for Direct Microscopic Detection of Parasites

Concentrated Wet Mounts

Concentrated wet mounts of blood, stool, or urine specimens can be examined microscopically for the presence of eggs, cysts, larvae, or vegetative cells of parasites.

Blood Smears

Blood smears for **sporozoan (malaria)** and **flagellate (trypanosome) parasites** are stained with Giemsa.

■ EXAMINATION OF PREPARED MATERIAL

The simple Gram stain or acid-fast stain is the fastest and least expensive method for presumptive diagnosis in these common clinical settings.

Two types of infection are important to distinguish: Infections caused by a *single species*, or **monomicrobial**, and infections caused by *multiple species*, or **polymicrobial**.

Infections caused by common single species or by classic infectious agents include *Streptococcus pneumoniae* pneumonia, *Staphylococcus aureus* abscesses or pyodermas, *H. influenzae* tracheobronchitis or meningitis in infants, *Clostridium perfringens* gas gangrene, *Nocardia* spp. lung abscesses, and gonococcal urethritis.

Polymicrobial presentations: Commonly encountered infections of this type are surgical wound (skin flora) infection, aspiration (oropharyngeal flora) pneumonia, perirectal (fecal flora) abscesses, and tubo-ovarian (vaginal flora) abscess.

■ SEARCH FOR MICROORGANISMS

After the full extent of the material has been examined on low power, a representative area should be selected for viewing with the oil immersion lens. A 40X or 60X lens is preferred for scanning, and a 100X lens is used for final evaluation.

Strict criteria for **microbial morphotypes** should be maintained. Organisms should be evaluated for shape, size, and Gram reaction. Because cell wall-damaged bacteria, antibiotic-treated bacteria, or dead bacteria may appear falsely Gram-negative, their shapes and sizes are critical "cocharacteristics."

- ❖ ***Examine more than one area of the smear:*** More than one organism should be found if possible.
- ❖ ***Do not overinterpret the findings:*** Specific diagnosis should be limited to a small number of instances in which the smear is classic in its presentation and the extent of infection is not an issue. If acid-fast bacteria are suspected, the acid-fast stain should be performed before an opinion is rendered. If a fungal element is not clearly Gram-positive, a calcofluor stain should be performed. Both of these follow-up stains can be performed on the decolorized, Gram-stained preparation.

KEY POINTS

- ❖ The microscopic examination of clinical specimens is used to detect bacterial cells, fungal elements, parasites (eggs, larvae, or adult forms), and viral inclusions present in infected cells.
- ❖ For bacteriology, the Gram and Ziehl-Neelsen stains are usually sufficient, but for the demonstration of fungi or parasites special stains or concentration techniques may be required.

IMPORTANT QUESTION

1. Describe identification of common microbes under the microscope.

MULTIPLE CHOICE QUESTIONS (MCQs)

1. Which of the following include the differential stains?
   a. Gram satin
   b. Acid-fast stain
   c. All of the above
   d. None of the above
2. Method(s) for detection for direct microscopic detection of parasite is/are:
   a. Concentrated wet mounts
   b. Blood smears for sporozoan (malaria)
   c. Blood smears for flagellate (trypanosome) parasites
   d. All of the above

ANSWERS

1. c   2. d

Index

Page numbers followed by *f* refer to figure, *b* refer to box, and *t* refer to table

■ A

Abiogenesis 4
Abortion 52
  spontaneous 50
Abscess 98
  purulent 48
Accessory sinuses, normal flora of 44
Acetone 211
Acid 158
  alcohol decolorizer 214
  anionic detergents 157
  fast
    bacilli 208, 212
    organisms 214, 222
    stain 208, 212, 222
  fuchsin 208
Acidic dyes 208
Acidic protoplasm 210
Acquired immunodeficiency syndrome 59, 87
Acridine dyes 159
Actinomycetes 52
Actinomycosis 52
Active immunity 105, 106, 106*t*, 108
  types of 106
Adenitis, mesenteric 57
Adhesion 88
African sleeping sickness 55
Agar gel precipitation test 140
Agar media 69
  types of 70*t*
Agglutination 138
  reaction 136, 137, 138*t*, 144
  applications of 138
Agglutinin 138
Agranulocytosis 126
Air filters 156
Albert's stain 215, 215*f*
Alcaligenes faecalis 29, 52
Alcohol 150, 157, 158, 160, 168, 211, 214
Aldehydes 150, 158, 159, 161, 169
Alkaline peptone water 71, 72
Alkalis 158
Allergens 122
Alpha-hemolytic streptococci 45
Amebae 55
Amies transport medium 73
Aminoglycosides 173
Amoebozoa 55
Ampholytic agents 168

Amphoteric agents 168
Anaerobic culture methods 75
Anaerobic media 72, 73
Anaerobiosis, methods of 75
Anaphylaxis 122
  mechanism of 123
  primary mediators of 124
  secondary mediators of 124
Anatomical waste, animal 182
Ancylostoma duodenale 56
Anemia, hemolytic 126
Aniline dyes 159
Anionic agents 159, 168
Anthrax 6, 8
Antibacterial drugs, mechanisms of action of 173*t*, 174
Antibiotic 10, 172, 177
  susceptibility testing 75
  therapy 51
  use for 157
Antibody 141
  dependent cell-mediated cytotoxicity 125
  reactions 136*b*
Antigen 123, 133, 141
  bacterial 75
  quantitative estimation of 137
  types of 136*b*
Antiglobulin test 138, 139*f*
  principle of 138
Antimicrobial agent 172, 173
Antimicrobial sensitivity testing 66
Antiseptics 11, 149, 173
Antisera 9, 119
Antistreptolysin-O test 140
Aperture diaphragm 198
Arenavirus complex, tacaribe group of 59
Arsphenamine 10
Arthritis 49, 51
  septic 49, 51
Arthropod-borne diseases 86
Arthus reaction 127
Asbestos filters 156
Ascaris lumbricoides 56
Ascoli's thermoprecipitin test 136, 137
Asepsis 81, 90, 166
  surgical 90, 166
Aspergillosis 54
Aspergillus fumigatus 54
Asphyxia 49
Athlete's foot 53

Atopic reactions, clinical expression of 125
Atopy 122, 125
   mechanism of 125
Auramine-rhodamine method 222
Autoclave 153
   components of 153
   cooling 154
   principle of 153
   tapes 155
Autoimmune diseases, classification of 133
Autoimmunity 132, 133
   cross reacting antigens theory of 133
   mechanisms of 132

■ B

Babesial infection 55
Babesiosis 55
Bacillary dysentery 50
Bacilli 21, 221
   arrangement 24
   gram-negative 221
   gram-positive 49, 221
Bacillus 28
   anthracis 8, 28, 49, 179
   Calmette-Guérin 112
   neisseria 211
   stearothermophilus 34, 155
   subtilis 152
Bacitracin 173
Backache 59
Bacteremia 49, 50, 53
   catheter-related 49
Bacteria 19, 20, 48, 48t, 52, 63, 142, 155
   aerobic 40
   anaerobic 40, 74
   arrangement of 23f
   capsulated 28
   concentration of 155
   direct microscopic detection of 220
   gram-negative 211
   gram-positive 25, 211
   isolating pure cultures of 7
   L-forms of 34
   microscopic examination of 7
   morphology of 19
   physiology of 37
   shape of 21, 22f
   size of 21
   study of 21
   traumatic inoculation of 52
   typing of 29
Bacterial cell
   anatomy of 24, 24f, 34
   arrangement of 22
   components 24
   wall
      chemical structure of 25f
      synthesis, inhibition of 173, 174

Bacterial cellular morphologies 221f
Bacterial cytoplasmic membrane function,
   inhibition of 173, 175
Bacterial flagellum, structure of 30f
Bacterial growth
   curve 38, 38f, 41
      phases of 38
   principle of 37
   spread of 30
Bacterial nucleic acid synthesis, inhibition
   of 173
Bacterial nucleus 31
Bacterial nutrition 39
Bacterial protein 160
   synthesis, inhibition of 173, 176
Bacterial spore 32, 32f, 155
Bacterial toxins 155
Bacterial vaccines 107, 112
Bacterial vaginosis 53
Bacteriology 10
   father of 7
Bacteriophages 75, 88
   separation of 155
Bacteroides fragilis 207
Balantidial dysentery 55
Balantidium coli 55
Bancroftian filariasis 56
Barber's itch 53
Basal body 29
Basal media 68, 69
Basic dyes 208, 214
Beef tapeworm 55
Benzoyl peroxide 163
Betadine 160, 164
Beta-lactam
   agents 174
   antibiotics 175
Binary fission 37
Biogroup aegyptius 51
Biomedical waste 179, 191
   categories of 180, 180b, 182t
   handlers 190
   management 179, 188
Biosafety 189
Biotechnology 184
Bipolaris 54
Birth 46
Bisphenols 157
Black piedra 54
Blastomyces dermatitidis 54, 64
Blastomycosis 54
Bleaching powder 160, 164
Blood 105
   agar 70, 73
   flukes 55
   smears 65, 223
Bloodstream 97
   infection, central line-associated 90

Index

Bordetella pertussis 52
Borrelia burgdorferi 52, 142
Borrelia recurrentis 52
Botulism 50
    infant 50
Brain abscesses 53
Brazilian purpuric fever 51
Breast milk 107
Bright-field microscope 195, 196
Bronchiolitis 58
Bronchitis 51, 58
Broth media 69
Browne's tube 152, 155
Brownian movement 206
Brucella melitensis 52
Brucellosis 52, 138
Burkholderia cepacia 51, 206
Burkholderia mallei 51, 207
Burkholderia pseudomallei 51, 206
Burkitt's lymphoma 57
Burns, severe 51

■ C

Calcium hypochlorite 164
California encephalitis virus 59, 60
Candida albicans 54
Capsular polysaccharides 112
Capsule
    functions of 29
    staining of 216
    swelling reaction 29
Carbapenems 175
Carbol fuchsin 208
Carbon dioxide 40
Carbuncles 48
Carcinoma
    hepatocellular 59
    nasopharyngeal 57
Cardiobacterium hominis 53
Carpet culture 75
Catalyst 76
Cell
    envelope 24, 25, 34
    gram-positive 210, 211
    interior 25, 31, 34
    membrane 158
    motility 27
    wall 24, 25
        defective organisms 34
        gram-negative 25, 26*f*
        gram-positive 26*f*
        integrity of 212
        protection of 29
        structure 211
Cellular appendages 24, 27
Cellulitis 49, 51
Central nervous system 51, 97

Cephalosporins 173, 174
Cerebral abscess 51
Cerebrospinal fluid 62, 97, 203, 220
Cervicitis 49
Cetrimide 160, 164
Chaga's disease 55
Chamber pressure 154
Chancroid 51
Chemical
    agents 150, 157, 159, 168
    control 155
    disinfection 187
    energy, generation of 27
    food preservatives 150, 158, 160, 168
    indicator 152
    liquid waste 183
    requirements 39
    sterilization 150, 158, 161, 169
    waste 183
Chemiluminescence-linked immunoassay 136, 141
Chemotherapeutic agents 172, 177
Chemotherapy 9
    antimicrobial 172
Chicken cholera vaccine 6
Chinese liver fluke 55
Chlamydia
    psittaci 53
    trachomatis 45, 53
Chlamydophila pneumoniae 53
Chloramines 160
    inorganic 160
    organic 160
Chloramphenicol 173, 176
Chlorhexidine 150, 159, 160, 164, 168
Chlorine 150, 160, 168
    dioxide 162
Chloroxylenol 150, 159, 160, 164, 168
Chocolate agar 70, 71
Cholera 8, 50
Chondrioids 31
Chorioretinitis 99
Chromobacterium violaceum 52, 206
Chromoblastomycosis 54
Chromosomal segregation, mediation of 27
Ciliophora 55
Cirrhosis 58
Clean technique 90, 166
Clonorchiasis 55
Clonorchis sinensis 55
Clostridium
    botulinum 50
    difficile 165
    perfringens 49, 140, 223
    tetani 40, 50, 206
Coagglutination 138, 139
Coccidioides immitis 54, 64, 179

Coccidioidomycosis 54
Cold acid-fast stain 222
Cold chain 113
   equipment 113
Cold sterilization 157
Colitis, hemolytic 50
Colorado tick fever virus 59, 60
Colostrum 107
Common cold 58, 59
Community infections 50
Complement fixation
   reactions 144
   test 136, 139
Complement system 105
Compound light microscope 196, 197*f*, 201
Confocal microscopy 195
Conjunctiva 98, 105
   normal flora of 43
Conjunctivitis 49, 51, 58
   purulent 51
Contact dermatitis 129
Convalescent serum 65
Cooked meat broth 73
Coombs' test 138, 139*f*
Core polysaccharide 27
Cornea 98
Corneal infections 50
Coronavirus 59, 60
Corynebacterium 43
   diphtheriae 24, 71, 140, 215
   xerosis 43
Coryza 58
Cotrimoxazole 177
Counterimmunoelectrophoresis 137
Coxsackievirus 57, 60
Cramps, abdominal 50
Cresol 150, 159, 168
Crimean congo hemorrhagic fever 59
Cross infection 84, 85
Cryptococcus neoformans 54, 64, 216
Cryptosporidiosis 55
Cryptosporidium 214, 222
Crystal violet-iodine complex 211
Culture methods 68, 74
Cutaneous basophil hypersensitivity 129
Cycloserine 173
Cystic fibrosis 51
Cystitis 50
Cytokines 125
Cytolytic reactions 125
Cytomegalovirus 56
Cytoplasm 25, 31
Cytoplasmic membrane 24, 27, 31
   functions of 27
Cytotoxic reactions 125
   drug-induced 126

■ D

Dapsone 173
Dark ground
   illumination 29
   microscope 203
Dengue
   fever 58
   hemorrhagic fever 127
   virus 58, 60
Deoxycholate citrate agar 70, 71
Deoxyribonucleic acid 25, 31
   single circular chromosome of 25
Dependovirus 57
Dermatophytosis 54
Diaminopyrimidines 177
Diarrhea 50, 57, 59
   antibiotic associated 50
   bloody 50
   infant 51, 58
   nonbloody 50
Dioxins 187
Diphtheria
   bacilli 136, 137
   cutaneous 49
Diphyllobothriasis 55
Diphyllobothrium latum 55
Direct immunofluorescence 141
Dirofilaria immitis 56
Disinfectant
   categories of 163, 164*b*
   low-level 164
Disinfection 11, 149, 156, 157, 157*t*, 163
   high-level 164
   methods of 149, 150*b*, 168
Disseminated infection, acute-onset 52
Dizziness 59
Doderlien's bacilli 46
Dog tapeworm 55
Donovania 53
Dry heat 150
   sterilization 151
Dry thermal treatment 187
Dwarf tapeworm 55
Dyes 159
Dysentery, amoebic 55

■ E

Ear infections 95, 99
Earthenware filters 155
Ebola virus 60
Echinococcosis 55
Echinococcus granulosus 55
Echoviruses 58, 60
Ecthyma gangrenosum 51
Eikenella corrodens 53
Electrolytes, elevated levels of 151

Index

Electron microscopy 28, 30, 31, 195
Elek test 136, 137
Elephantiasis 56
Empyema 49
Encephalitis 58, 59
Endocarditis 49, 51, 53
Endospore 32, 34
Endotoxin 27, 88, 89, 89*t*
Enriched media 69-72, 77
Entamoeba histolytica 55, 142
Enteritis 50
Enterobius vermicularis 56
Enzyme-linked fluorescent immunoassay 136, 141
Enzyme-linked immunosorbent assay 65, 136, 141
    types of 141, 142*f*
    uses of 142, 142*t*
Eosinophil chemotactic factor 124
Epidermophyton floccosum 54
Epiglottis 95
Epiglottitis 51
Epstein-Barr virus 57
Equine encephalitis virus 58, 60
Erysipelas 49
Erysipelothrix rhusiopathiae 52
Erythrovirus 57
Escherichia coli 50, 142, 206, 210*f*, 211
Etest strip 66
Ethanol 150, 160, 168
Ethyl alcohol 150, 160, 164, 168
Ethylene oxide 150, 158, 159, 162
Eukaryotes 20
Eukaryotic cells 20, 20*t*
Eulenozoa 55
Exophiala 54
Exosporium 33
Exotoxins 88, 89, 89*t*
Exserohilum 54
External ear 43
Eye
    infections 57, 95, 98
    lens antigen of 133
Eyeball, infections of 99

■ F

Falciparum malaria 62
Fasciola hepatica 55
Fascioliasis 55
Febrile illness, mild 58
Feces 95
Fetus, intrauterine infection of 52
Fever 50, 51, 58, 59, 105
    enteric 50
    mountain 59
    paratyphoid 50
    pontiac 51
    relapsing 52

    rheumatic 49
    scarlet 49
    virus, hemorrhagic 59, 60
Filariasis 56
Filoviridae 60
Filtration 150, 155
Fimbria 31
    demonstration of 31
Fish tapeworm 55
Flagella 29
    arrangement of 30*f*
    demonstration of 29
Flash method 152
Flaviviridae 58, 60
Flavobacterium menigosepticum 207
Flocculation 136
    tests 136
Fluids, supercritical 150, 158, 162, 169
Fluorescent microscopy 195
Follicular conjunctivitis, acute 57
Folliculitis 48
Fonsecaea pedrosoi 54
Food 86
    poisoning 49
Foodborne botulism 50
Forespore 32
Formaldehyde 150, 159, 161
    gas 161
Fosfomycin 173
Francisella tularensis 51, 179
Frank encephalitis 58
Fried egg appearance 34
Fungal
    agents 54
    cultures 64
    disease, classification of 54*t*
    infections 53, 64
    serology 64
Fungi 19, 43, 53, 64, 86
    direct microscopic detection of 217, 222
Fungus 222
    infections 54
Furazolidone 176
Fusidic acid 173

■ G

Gaffkya tetragena 23*f*
Gardnerella vaginalis 53, 207
Gas gangrene 86
Gaseous sterilants 150, 158, 169
Gas-liquid chromatography 66
Gastric adenocarcinoma 50
Gastritis 50
Gastroenteritis 50, 59
    epidemic viral 59
    infant 52

Index

Gastrointestinal tract 51, 95, 104
  normal flora of 45
Gell and Coombs classification 122
Genital infections 96
Genital tract 96
Genitalia 43
Genitourinary tract 104
  normal flora of 45
Germination 33
Giardia
  intestinalis 55
  lamblia 55
Giardiasis 55
Giemsa staining 63
Glassware 151, 152, 185
Glomerulonephritis, acute 49
Glottis 95
Glucose broth 72
Glutaraldehyde 150, 159, 161, 164
Glycogen 31
Glycopeptides 175
Gram stain 28, 34, 208, 210*f*, 208, 216, 219, 220
  interpretation of 209
  mechanism 210
  procedure 210*f*
  reactions 221*f*
Gram's method 211
Gramicidin 173
Granuloma inguinale 53
Granulomatis 53
Growth
  media, phases of 68, 69
  microbial 40
Guillain-Barre syndrome 50

■ H

Haemophilus
  ducreyi 51
  influenzae 28, 51, 97, 112, 138, 142
Hahn test 137
Halogens 150, 158-160, 168
Hand-foot-and-mouth disease 57
Hanging drop
  method 7
  preparation 203, 204, 204*f*, 205*f*
Hanta virus 59, 60
Hashimoto's thyroiditis 133
Headache 59
Healthcare waste 181
Heart 49
  muscle antigens 133
Heartworm 56
Heat 150
  application of 212
  sensitive
    materials 151
    solutions 155

Heavy metals 158-160, 168
  derivatives 150
Helicobacter pylori 50
Helminthes 55*t*
Hemagglutination test 31, 138, 139
Hemolytic disease 126
Hemolytic uremic syndrome 50
Heparin 124
Hepatitis 58
  A virus 58, 60
  acute 58, 59
  B 57, 119
    virus 94, 113
  C virus 58, 60
  cirrhosis, chronic 59
  E virus 59
  infectious 58
  serum 57
Herd immunity 108
  high-level of 109
Herpangina 57
Herpes viruses 56
Hexachlorophene 150, 159, 160, 168
Histamine 124
Histoplasma capsulatum 54, 64
Histoplasmosis 54
Hodgkin's disease 57
Hookworm disease 56
Hormones 150
Hortaea werneckii 54
Hospital infection 51
  control of 11, 90
  diagnosis of 11, 90
Host 83
Hot air
  oven, uses of 152
  sterilizer 151
Human body, normal microbial flora of 43
Human diseases 48, 48*t*, 53, 55, 55*t*, 56*t*, 57*t*, 58
Human immunodeficiency virus 59, 60, 65, 94, 160
Human infection, forms of 52
Human papilloma virus vaccine 113
Human T-cell leukemia virus 59, 60
Human tetanus immunoglobulin 119
Hyaluronidase 88
Hybrid virus vaccines 113
Hydrochloric acid 214
Hydrogen peroxide 150, 159, 162
Hymenolepiasis 55
Hymenolepis nana 55
Hypersensitivity 121, 122*t*, 125, 126, 126*f*, 127, 129
  cell mediated 128*f*
  delayed 122, 127, 128
  immediate 122
  reactions 121, 123*t*
    classification of 121

Hypochlorite 160, 168
  solution 160

I

Immune
  complex 127
    mediated disease, models of 127
  system 103
Immunity 9, 81, 103
  acquired 105
  active 105, 106, 106*t*, 108
  artificial
    active 106
    passive 107
  herd 108
  innate 103, 105
  instant 107
  local 108
  natural 103
    active 106
    passive 107
  nonspecific 104
  passive 106, 106*t*, 107
  specific 104
  types of 105
Immunization 9, 108, 114
  active 114, 119
  passive 114, 118, 119
  schedules 114
Immunoblotting techniques 136, 143
Immunochromatographic test 136
Immunodiffusion tests, types of 136
Immunoelectronmicroscopic tests 136, 143
Immunoelectrophoresis 136, 137, 144
Immunoenzyme test 143
Immunoferritin test 143
Immunofluorescence 136, 140, 144
  indirect 141
Immunoglobulin 111, 118
Immunology 10, 101
  father of 9
Immunoprophylaxis 111
Impetigo 48, 49
Incineration 151, 181
Incinerator
  advantage of 187
  disadvantages of 187
  types of 181
India ink preparation procedure 216
Indirect agglutination test 138, 139
Industrial eye injuries 51
Industrial methylated spirit 214
Inertization 188
Infection 3, 79, 81, 82, 84
  atypical 84, 85
  chain of 82, 83*f*
  classification of 83, 84*t*

control
  committee 91
  doctor 11
  nurse 11
  policy 91
  team 91
cutaneous 48, 51
diagnosis of 10
genitourinary 52
healthcare-associated 84, 90, 165
hospital associated 91
iatrogenic 84, 85
modes of transmission of 86, 91
mycotic 53
nosocomial 50, 53, 85
opportunistic 51, 52
primary 54*t*, 83, 84
route of 89
secondary 84
sources of 85, 90, 91
subclinical 84, 85
treatment of 10
zoonotic 50
Infectious agent 48, 82
Infectious disease 82
  types of 89
Inflammation 105, 127
Influenza 58, 113
  immunization 108
  virus
    A 58 60
    B 58, 60
    C 58, 60
Ingestion 87, 91
Inhalation 86, 91
Innate immunity 103, 105
  mechanisms of 104
Inoculation 87, 91
Insects 86, 87
Intestinal infections 52
Intestine, small 104
Intracytoplasmic inclusions 31
Intraocular structures 98
Intussusception 57
Iodine 150, 160, 168
Iodophor 164
  povidone-iodine 160
Ionizing radiation 156
Iritis 99
Isoniazid 173
Isopropyl alcohol 150, 160, 168

J

Jacuzzi rash 51
Jaundice 59
Jones-Mote reaction 129
Junin and Machupo viruses 60

K

Kahn test 136
Kala azar 55
Keratitis, amoebic 55
Keratoconjunctivitis, epidemic 57
Kidneys 49
Kinyoun method 222
Kirby-Bauer method 66
Klebsiella pneumoniae 50, 206
Koch's phenomenon 8
Koch's postulates 8, 8*f*, 9*b*
    limitations of 9

L

La Crosse virus 60
Laboratory infections 91
Lacrosse virus 59
Lactophenol cotton blue stain 217, 222
Lag phase 38, 39
Lancefield technique 136, 137
Land disposal 188
Lassa fever virus 59, 60
Latex agglutination test 138, 139
Lawn culture 74, 75
Legionella pneumophila 51
Legionnaires' disease 51, 65
Leishmania donovani 55
Leprosy 52
Leptospira interrogan 52
Leptospirosis 52
Leptotrichia buccalis 207
Leukemia, adult T-cell 59
Leukotrienes 125
Lid 153, 154
    margins 98
Light 40
    microscopy 195, 196
        methods of use of 198
        principle of 196
Lincosamides 173
Lipopolysaccharide 25-27
Lipoprotein 25, 26
Liquid
    culture 74
    media 69
        types of 72*t*
Listeria monocytogenes 52
Live attenuated
    anthrax vaccine 6
    microorganisms 106
Local immune complex disease 127
Loeffler's methylene blue 214
Loeffler's serum slope 70, 71
Lowenstein and Jensen medium 71
Lower respiratory tract disease 51, 96
Low-power objective 199, 205
Lung
    abscesses 53
    fluke 55
Lyme disease 52
Lymphadenitis 51, 52
Lymphocytic choriomeningitis virus 59, 60
Lymphoma, adult T-cell 59

M

MacConkey agar 70, 72, 73
Machupo viruses 59
Macrolides 173
Madurella mycetomatis 54
Magic bullet 10
Malachite green 212
Malaise 51
Malaria 55
Mancini method 137
Marburg virus 60
Mast cell 124*f*
McIntosh and Fildes anaerobic jar 75, 76*f*, 77
Measles 58
    atypical 58
    virus 58, 60
Media, classification of 68, 69*b*
Medical asepsis 90, 166
Membrane filters 156
Meningitis 49-53
    aseptic 57-59
    neonatal 50, 52
    pyogenic 62
    tubercular 52
Meningoencephalitis 49
Meningosepticum 52
Mercuric chloride 168
Mesosomes 25, 31
    functions of 31
Metabolic antagonism 173, 177
Metallic body implants 185
Metamonada 55
Methicillin-resistant *Staphylococcus aureus* 165
Methylene blue 76, 208, 212, 214
Microaerophilic organisms 40
Microbes 195
    study of 62
Microbial antagonisms 105
Microbial morphotypes 223
Microbiology 184
    branches of 10
    father of 14
    historical development of 3
    scientific development of 5
    scope of 10
Microorganisms 17, 19, 81
    control of 147

Index

destruction of 147
discovery of 4
first observation of 4
search for 223
Microscope 195
   care of 200
   parts of 196
Microscopy 34, 62, 195, 201
Microsporum canis 86
Microwave irradiation 188
Middle ear, tuberculosis of 52
Miliary tuberculosis 52
Milk, pasteurization of 152
Modern surgery, father of 7
Moist heat 150-153
Moisture 40
Molecular methods 65
Monobactams 175
Mononucleosis, infectious 57
Moraxella
   catarrhalis 44
   lacunata 44
Morganella morganii 206
Morphology 203
Motility 203
Mouth
   cavity 104
   normal flora of 44
Mucopolysaccharide 104
Mucormycosis 54
Mucous membrane 104
Multifocal pneumonia, life-threatening 51
Multiple organs 50
Mumps 58
   virus 58, 60
Mupirocins 173
Muscle
   ache 59
   weakness 58
Musculoskeletal system 51
Myalgia 59
   epidemic 57
Mycetoma 54
Mycobacteria 63
   atypical 52, 214, 222
Mycobacterium
   bovis 214, 222
   leprae 52, 214, 222
   smegmatis 45
   tuberculosis 71, 179, 211, 213, 214, 222
Mycolic acid 212
Mycology 10
Mycoplasma 22, 52, 63, 64
   pneumonia 52, 64
Mycosis 54
   types of 54
Myonecrosis 49
Myositis, suppurative 49

N

Nagler's reaction 140
Nail bed, infection of 51
Nalidixic acid 175
Nasopharynx, normal flora of 44
National Immunization Schedule 114, 115*t*
Nausea 50, 59
Necator americanus 56
Neck pain 59
Necrotizing fasciitis 49
Necrotizing pneumonia 51
Needle-mount method 217
Neisseria
   catarrhalis 23*f*
   gonorrhoeae 49
   meningitides 28, 112, 113, 138
Nematoda 56
Neoantigens 133
Neoplastic diseases 51
Nervous system 49
Neutralization tests 136, 140
Neutrophil chemotactic factors 124
Nitrates 150, 158, 160
Nitrites 150, 158, 160
Nitrofurantoin 176
Nitroimidazoles 173, 176
Nocardia
   asteroids 214, 222
   brasiliensis 214, 222
Nomenclature 19
Non-lactose fermenter 73
Norwalk virus 59, 60
Nose, normal flora of 44
Nosocomial pneumonia, cause of 51
Novobiocin 173, 176
Nucleic acid 66, 159
   synthesis, inhibitor of 175
Nutrient
   agar 69, 70
   broth 69, 72

O

O antigen 27
Oil-immersion
   lens 201
   objective 199
Oncoviruses, animal 60
Opsonization 136, 140
Optical system 196
Oral cavity 95, 104
Orbit, infections of 99
Ordinary pili 31
Organic acids 150, 158, 160
Organisms 206
   isolation of 155
Ornithosis 53

Orthomyxoviridae 58, 60
Ortho-phthalaldehyde 150
Osmotic effect 41
Osteomyelitis 49
Otitis 51
    externa 50
    media 49
Ouchterlony immune-double-diffusion technique 136, 137
Outer membrane 25, 26
Oxidative damage 150
Oxygen 40, 158, 162, 169
    peroxygens, forms of 150
Ozone 150, 163

■ P

Pain, abdominal 59
Panencephalitis, subacute sclerosing 58
Papillomavirus 57
Papovaviruses 57
Pappataci fever 59
Parabasala 55
Paracoccidioides brasiliensis 54
Paracoccidioidomycosis 54
Paragonimiasis 55
Paragonimus westermanni 55
Parainfluenza virus 58, 60
Paramyxoviridae 58, 60
Paranasal sinuses 95
Parasites 55, 55t, 65, 81, 86, 142
    direct microscopic detection of 223
Parasitology 10
Parvoviruses 57
Passive agglutination test 138, 139
Passive immunity 106, 106t, 107
    advantage of 107
Passive immunization 114, 118, 119
    indications of 108
Pasteurella multocida 51
Pasteurization 6, 152
Pathogenicity 81, 87
Pathogens 55, 81
    opportunist 82
    primary 82
    types of 82
Paul-Bunnell test 138
Pelvic inflammatory disease 49
Penicillinase 177
Penicillins 173, 174
Penicilliosis 54
Penicillium
    marneffei 54
    notatum 10
Peptic ulcers 50
Peptidoglycan 25
    smaller amount of 211
Peptone water 72

Peracetic acid 150, 163
Periodontal disease, severe 53
Peritoneal cavities 98
Peritonitis 51
Pernasal swab 95
Peroxyacetic acid 150, 163
Peroxygens 150, 158, 162, 169
pH 40
Phaeohyphomycosis 54
Phagocytosis 29
Pharyngitis 49, 57, 58
    vesicular 57
Pharyngoconjunctival fever 57
Phase-contrast microscope 195, 203
Phenol 150, 157, 159, 168, 212
    derivatives 159
Phenolic 150, 157, 159, 168
    compounds 158
Phialophora verrucosa 54
Photophobia 59
Picornaviridae 60
Piedraia hortae 54
Pili 31
    functions of 31
Pilins 31
Pinworm 56
    feotalism 56
Pityriasis versicolor 54
Plague 51
Plasma
    membrane 24, 27
    sterilization 150, 158, 162, 169
Plasmids 32, 88
    fingerprinting 66
    functions of 32
Plasmodium
    falciparum 55
    malariae 55
    ovale 55
    vivax 55
Platelet activating factor 124
Platyhelminthes 55
Pneumonia 49, 50, 52, 53, 57, 58
    primary
        atypical 52
        community-acquired 50
    ventilator-associated 90
Polio 57
Poliomyelitis immunization 108
Poliovirus 57, 60
Polyarthritis, epidemic 58
Polyclonal B-cell activation 133
Polymerase chain reaction 65
Polymicrobial 223
Polymyxins 173
Polyomavirus 57
Polyphosphate 31
Polysaccharide 27

Polyvinyl chloride 187
Pork tapeworm 55
Postdiphtheritic paralysis 49
Poststreptococcal glomerulonephritis 127
Potassium
    hydroxide 222
    hydroxide preparation 217, 222
    tellurite medium 71
Pour-plate culture 74
Precipitation 135
    reactions 135, 136
    uses of 136
Pressure filtration 156
Proctitis 49, 50
Prokaryotes 20
Prokaryotic cells 20, 20*t*
Propionibacterium 43
Prostaglandin 125
Prostate 50
    per rectum, massage of 97
Prostatitis 50, 97
Proteases 124
Proteins 151, 159
    acute phase 105
    denaturation 150
    subunits 112
Protoplasm 210
Protozoan diseases 140
Providencia stuartii 206
Pseudallescheria boydii 54
Pseudomembranous colitis 50
Pseudomonas aeruginosa 44, 50, 206
Psittacosis 53
Puberty 46
Pulmonary disease 51
Purified protein derivative 128
Pyelonephritis 50
Pyogenic infections 49, 50

■ Q

Quaternary ammonium compounds 150, 157, 159
Quellung reaction 29
Quinolones 173, 175

■ R

Rabbit fever 51
Rabies 59, 113, 119
    vaccine 6
    virus 59, 60
Radiation 150, 156
Radioimmunoassay 136, 141
Rapid tests 136, 143
Rat bite fever 53
Renal syndrome 59
Reoviridae 59, 60
Reservoir hosts 85, 86

Respiratory diseases 57
Respiratory enzymes 31
Respiratory infection 49, 57
Respiratory syncytial virus 58, 60
Respiratory system, infarctions of 51
Respiratory tract
    infections 51
    syndromes 58
Retroviridae 59, 60
Reversed passive agglutination 139
Rhabdoviridae 59, 60
Rheumatoid arthritis 127, 133
Rhinovirus 58, 60
Ribosomes 25, 31
Rickettsia 63
    rickettsiae 53
Rifamycins 173, 176
Ring test 136, 137
Robertson's cooked meat broth 72
Rocket electrophoresis 137
Rocky mountain spotted fever 53
Rose-Waaler test 138
Ross river virus 58, 60
Rotavirus 59, 60
Roundworm 56
Rubella 58
    virus 58, 60

■ S

Sabia viruses 59
Safranin counterstain 209
Salmonella typhi 112
Salpingitis 49
Salvarsan 10
Sandfly fever virus 59, 60
Sanitary landfills 188
Saprophytes 81
Scalded skin syndrome 49
Schick test 140
Schistosomiasis 55
Screw-feed technology 187
Seitz filter 156
Selenite F broth 71, 72
Semisolid agar 30
Semliki forest virus 58, 60
Sendai virus 60
Sepsis 51
Septicemia 49-52
Serological methods 28
Serological tests 135
    principle of 135
    uses of 135
Serology 65
Serotherapy 9
Serotonin 124
Serum sickness 127
Severe acute respiratory syndrome 59

Sex pili 31
Sexually transmitted disease 51, 53
Shake culture 74
Shanghai fever 51
Sheep liver fluke 55
Shigella dysenteriae 50
Shigellosis 50
Shock, anaphylactic 123
Shwartzman reaction 129
Silkworm, Pebrine disease of 5
Silver nitrate 168
Sindbis virus 58, 60
Sintered glass filters 156
Sinusitis 49, 51, 53
Skin 104
    candidiasis of 54
    lesions 51
    normal flora of 43
    tuberculosis of 52
Slide
    agglutination 138
    flocculation test 136, 137
    test 136, 137
Smallpox virus 56
Smear 207
    preparation 207
Sodium hypochlorite 164
Soft sore 51
Soft tissue infections 49
Sonic stresses 41
Sore
    eyes 59
    throat 59
South American hemorrhagic fever 59
Spasm 58
Spaulding's classification 167, 167t
Special capsule staining techniques 28
Special staining methods 29
Sperm antigens 133
Spermine 104
Spirilla 22
Spirochetes 22, 52
Spontaneous generation 4
    disapproved theory of 6
Spore 32, 90, 166
    coat 33
    cortex 33
    physiology of 33
    septum 32
    shape of 33
    staining of 216
    types of 33f
    uses of 34
Sporothrix schenckii 54
Sporotrichosis 54
Sputum 96
St. Louis encephalitis virus 58, 60
Stab culture 74
Staining methods 203, 207, 220

Staphylococcus
    aureus 20, 48, 139, 223
    epidermidis 43, 46
    saprophyticus 176
Steam sterilizers, types of 154
Sterile technique 90, 166, 167
Sterilization 11, 149, 151, 157t, 162
    control 34, 152
    fractional 152
    intermittent 153
    methods of 149, 150b, 168
    techniques 6
Stiffness 59
Stillbirth 52
Stomach aspiration 96
Streak culture 74, 74f
Streptobacillus moniliformis 53
Streptococcal pharyngitis 49
Streptococcal toxic shock syndrome 49
Streptococci, grouping of 136, 137
Streptococcus
    moniliformis 207
    pneumoniae 28, 49, 112, 138, 211, 220, 223
    pyogenes infection 49, 140
Streptogramins 173
Stroke culture 74
Strongyloides stercoralis 56
Strongyloidiasis 56
Stuart's transport medium 73
Subunit vaccine 112
Sugar media 69, 73
Sulfonamides 173, 177
Sulfuric acid 213, 214
Superkingdoms system 19
Suppressor T-cells 133
Surgical instruments 161
Surgical site infections 51, 90
Swabs
    nasopharyngeal 95
    pharyngeal 96
    postnasal 95
    rectal 96
Syphilis 52, 136, 137
    diagnosis of 140, 141
Systemic candidiasis 54
Systemic immune complex disease 127
Systemic lupus erythematosus 127

■ T

Taenia
    saginata 55
    solium 55
Taeniasis 55
Teichoic acid 25
Test tubes 151
Tetanus 50
    spore of 86

Index

Tetracyclines 173, 176
Tetrads 24
Tetrathionate broth 71, 72
Thermocouples 152, 155
Thicker peptidoglycan cell wall 211
Thioglycolate broth 73
Threadworm 56
Thrombocytopenic purpura 126
Tick fever 59
Tinea nigra 54
Tissue 105
    damage 127
    deep subcutaneous 49
Togaviridae 58, 60
Toluidine blue 214
Toxic shock syndrome 49
Toxigenicity test 88, 140
Toxin neutralization 140
Toxoid 112
    inactivated 106
Toxoplasma gondii 55
Toxoplasmosis 55
Trachoma 53
Transfusion reactions 125
Transport media 69, 73, 77
Treponema pallidum 52, 97
    hemagglutination 138
Trichina worm 56
Trichinella spiralis 56
Trichinosis 56
Trichomonas 97
    vaginalis 55
Trichophyton verrucosum 86
Trichuriasis 56
Trichuris trichiura 56
Trimethoprim 173
Trypanosoma
    brucei 55
    cruzi 55
Tube agglutination
    test 138
    uses of 138
Tube flocculation test 136, 137
Tube test 136, 137
Tuberculosis 8, 52
    disseminated 52
    pulmonary 52
Tularemia 51
Tyndallization 153
Typhoid fever 50
Typhus fevers 138
Tyrocidine 173

■ U

United Nations Conference on
    Environment and Development
    189

Universal Child Immunization 114
Universal Immunization Program 113, 114
Upper respiratory tract
    infection 58, 95, 104
    normal flora of 44
Ureaplasma urealyticum 46
Urethral discharge 96
Urethritis 49
Urinary tract infections 50-52, 96
    catheter-associated 90
    nosocomial 51
Urine, normal flora of 104

■ V

Vaccines 106, 111, 115-118, 157
    conjugates 106
    inactivated 112
    killed 112
    live 112
    preparation of 161
    types of 112
Vacuoles 25
Vacuum 156
Vaginal swab, high 96
Vaginitis, protozoal 55
Valley fever 54
Vancomycin 173
Varicella zoster virus 56
Varicose ulcers 50
Venereal disease research laboratory test
    136, 137
Vesicular stomatitis virus 60
Vibrio 22
    cholerae 29, 50, 89, 206
Violet dye 209
Viral components 112
Viral neutralization 140
Viral vaccines 107, 112
Virology 10
Virulence 87
    determinants of 87
    factor 29
Viruses 56, 58, 59, 64, 142
    discovery of 9
    isolation 155
    killed 111
    live 111
Vomiting 50, 59

■ W

Waste
    contaminated 184
    hazardous 180
    human anatomical 182
    infectious 180
    management program 189

non-infectious hazardous 180
   segregation 180, 191
   soiled 182
   treatment 181
   types of 180*b*, 182
Water 154
Weil-Felix reaction 138
Western blot 143
Wet coverslip preparation 203
Wet mounts 62, 65, 203, 220, 223
   direct examination of 220
Wet thermal treatment 187
Wheezing 58
Whipworm 56
Whirlpool rash 51
White fluids 159
White piedra 54
Whooping cough 52
Wilson and Blair medium 73
Wound 98
   botulism 50
   infections of 50, 95
Wuchereria bancrofti 56

■ Y

Yeasts 43, 220
Yellow fever 58
   virus 58, 60
Yersinia 28
   pestis 28, 51

■ Z

Ziehl-Neelsen
   reagents 214
   stain 34, 62, 208, 212, 213*f*, 219
     modified 34
Zinc 104
Zoonosis 85
Zoonotic diseases 86
Zygomycosis 54